TOO LITTLE S ANNOYING SYN

Cramp, headaches, nervousness, shaky hands, insomnia, frequent urination, feeling 'not quite with it', fainting, craving salty snacks, swollen ankles, biting fingernails, PMT, stress related conditions, and 'the worried well'.

by
Sally Gething
© Sally Gething 2012

With thanks to

Russell Stark,

who gave me sea salt when I was ill.

CONTENTS

l) Feeling World-weary

m) Period Pain/PMT

n) Teenage Girls

o) The Menopause

p) Swollen Ankles

q) Biting Fingernails

r) Recovering from a Shock, an Asthma Attack, a Panic Attack, a Hyperventilation Attack, or any Fainting or Collapsing for an Unknown Reason

s) Craving Crisps, Nuts, and Other Salty or Spicy Foods

t) Stress, or any Conditions Made Worse by Stress

5 But What If I Have These Symptoms as well as an Existing Health Problem?

i) Already Taking Medication

ii) Blood Pressure Problems

iii) Common Questions about Blood Pressure

iv) Diabetes

1
INTRODUCTION

I first came across the health benefits of sea salt in 1999 when I was suddenly taken ill. I was unable to recover on my own and was given a hot drink containing sea salt to see if it would help. It was amazing. Within five minutes I felt normal. I was able to jump in my car straight away and make the forty minute drive home without any problems at all. At this point I had been ill with M.E. for ten years, and had found very few remedies that actually helped me. I went on to suffer from M.E. for another ten years, and sea salt became a major part of my health weaponry. It worked!

But this book isn't all about M.E., nor is it about my health and recovery. In my professional capacity as an Alternative

Health Practitioner, I have recommended adding sea salt to the diets of hundreds of people. All but a very small number of them found it to be of such benefit that they haven't stopped using sea salt since, and some of them have been kind enough to share their own experiences in this book.

In fact it was these people who asked me to write this book, because they found it difficult to explain to other people why they were taking sea salt and what its health benefits were.

Over the last ten years, hundreds of my clients have asked me all sorts of questions about sea salt, table salt, blood pressure, their own health problems, where to get the salt from, how to take it, how much to take, and how to know when they've have had enough. All of those questions, and more, are answered in this book.

To begin with I'll tell you what sea salt is and how it can help (often in less than twenty minutes) with a number of complaints, from headaches and hangovers, to sleeplessness, nervousness, shaky hands, frequent urination, and cramp. You might be surprised just how many ailments sea salt can help with! Later, I'll go into a little more detail and show how people with longer-term medical problems, such as high blood pressure, diabetes, and asthma, can add sea salt to their diets, and monitor what effects, if any, it has had on their health.

I hope you enjoy reading this book and I hope you benefit, as I have, by introducing sea salt to your diets.

2
THE CONNECTION BETWEEN THE BUTEYKO METHOD AND SEA SALT

When I decided to write this book many people asked how I knew so much about sea salt. Well, for the answer, I have to take you back to the 1990s, and to an episode of the documentary TV programme Q.E.D. showing a new approach to controlling asthma. The method was called the Buteyko Method, and it involved teaching people to control their asthma symptoms with their breathing rather than medication. The originator of the method, a Russian doctor called Konstantin Pavlovich Buteyko, proposed that if an asthmatic got their breathing rate back to normal, that is between 4 and 6 litres of air per minute (at rest), then most of their symptoms would decrease dramatically. As most people with asthma breathe about 15 to 20 litres of air a minute, he came up with a variety of breathing exercises to reduce the overall rate. Most people who learn this method are able to reduce their medication and have a better quality of life.

I immediately knew I wanted to train to teach this method, and eventually discovered a husband and wife team, Russell and Jennifer Stark, who train other teachers and had taught the Buteyko Method to over 5000 asthmatics in Australia and New Zealand. I began my training and discovered there were two parts to the method. One involved retraining the breathing; the other was the importance of minerals to the human body. As sea salt contains vast amounts of minerals, adding it to your diet gives you the minerals you need.

Over the next ten years I taught the method to over 500 people, and advised all of them how they could normalise their mineral levels by adding sea salt to their diets. Most of my clients were amazed that I was telling them to eat salt – after all, they had come to me to learn how to breathe normally. However, virtually every single one tried the sea salt, and a huge majority continued to use it. After all, it makes sense: why wouldn't you want the correct level of minerals in your body?

3
WHAT HAPPENS TO THE MINERAL LEVELS WHEN A BODY IS UNDER STRESS?

When the human body is under stress, it enters the state commonly known as 'fight or flight'. The heart rate increases, the digestion slows, less saliva is produced, and the liver releases sugar to quickly provide energy. The automatic breathing pattern increases and too much carbon dioxide is breathed out. Although carbon dioxide is often seen as the waste gas of breathing, it needs to maintain a certain level to regulate bodily functions. If the carbon dioxide levels are too low, the blood becomes more alkaline than is healthy. To prevent this from happening, and to get the body back into homeostasis, which means 'balance', the kidneys begin to dump bicarbonate ions.

The kidneys cannot dump bicarbonate ions on their own, so they dump minerals such as potassium, calcium, magnesium and phosphates as well. This results in depleted mineral levels, with those minerals being excreted in urine. In other words, when our bodies are under stress we lose minerals.

We can look at it in the short term and long term.

Short Term – The Stress of a Shock

Someone has nearly bashed into your car. This is a shock, and there are numerous ways your body might have reacted to it. Maybe your palms became sweaty. Maybe you felt you needed to take a deep breath, or a number of deep breaths. You may have noticed your hands, or even your whole body, shaking. Or you might have simply felt shaken up, faint, or woozy. The stress of this situation will have caused your body to dump minerals, and the symptoms that follow can take seconds to manifest. You will, more than likely, need to recover in some way, by having a short rest, a drink, a lie down, or by eating something. You probably will have fully recovered within 24 hours.

An easy solution to speed up your recovery by replacing the minerals your body will have lost is to have one of the sea salt drinks as soon as possible, or to have a hot bath with a handful of sea salt dissolved in it, or by adding a bit of extra sea salt to your meals that day.

Long Term – Prolonged Stress

If you are under stress for prolonged periods, let's say six months, as you deal with a family problem, or have to do extra work, or have your daily living routine disrupted by forces outside of your control (etc.), your mineral levels will be constantly reduced. This could affect your whole body and, in turn, your daily life. You may be very tired, irritable, have symptoms that plague you from time to time, such as stomach irregularities, headaches or poor sleep patterns. In essence, you'll be feeling below par, exhausted, and not in the best of health. You may be aware your poor state of health is due to stress, but if there is no way of stopping it, you may have no other option than to learn to live with it. But you don't need to, because many of these symptoms may be remedied by adding sea salt to your diet on a daily basis.

4
THE SYMPTOMS SEA SALT CAN HELP WITH

People are amazed when I tell them what can be cured or made better by simply adding sea salt to their diets. In this section I'll take you through the five most common symptoms a diet lacking in minerals can cause, and show you the quick and easy ways to alleviate them. If you have two or more of the following list, then your diet is probably too low in salt/minerals.

The five main symptoms are:

1 Cramp
2 Headaches (this section includes hangovers and migraines)

3 Nervousness and panic attacks (this section includes shaky hands and anticipating a big day ahead)

4 Sleeplessness, insomnia and waking in the night

5 Frequent urination

Over the last twelve years I have also linked lack of salt/minerals to other situations and conditions. If you recognise any of the list below, lack of salt/minerals may have an important role to play, and the simple act of adding sea salt to your food could solve the problem or help you recover and get back to normal.

1 Feeling 'not quite with it'
2 Feeling world-weary
3 Period pain, premenstrual tension, and the menopause
4 Swollen ankles
5 Biting fingernails
6 Recovering from a shock, an asthma attack, a panic attack, a hyperventilation attack, or any fainting or collapsing for an unknown reason
7 Craving crisps, nuts and other salty snacks
8 Stress, or any condition made worse by stress

There are many ways to add sea salt to your diet as a way of alleviating these symptoms: you can drink it, nibble it, bathe in it, or cook with it. For a full explanation of all of these methods, read Chapter 8: How To Take Sea Salt.

Of course, if you've been advised by a health care professional to reduce your intake of salt, or if you're taking medication, talk to a doctor before increasing your intake of sea salt.

a) Cramp

Cramp is often felt in the legs or the hands, and most commonly at night. There are lots of old wives' tales about how to get rid of cramp, such as sleeping with a brown paper bag under the sheets, taking quinine, and drinking tonic water, among others, but an easy, cheap and efficient way to rid yourself of cramp is to simply have some sea salt.

For some of us, cramp, although very painful, is a minor problem that only affects us once or twice a year. But for others, it can happen on such a regular basis that it can disturb our sleep night after night. Once we are in a pattern of sleepless nights, it can affect our whole life, as we become sleepy and lethargic during the day. In fact, it can make us feel particularly unwell. It can affect our routines, hobbies, friends and quality of life. We can often feel a lot older, and more weary, than we did before.

Sometimes cramp is a result of an illness, or the taking of medication. Sometimes people have no idea why they get cramp, or how to get rid of it. Many of us will not consult a doctor about it, as it seems such an 'unimportant' problem.

As I said earlier, taking sea salt is an effective way of treating cramp. You can either treat the symptom and just nibble some sea salt when you get an attack, or you can take sea salt on a more regular basis as a preventative measure, so that you don't get the cramp symptoms at all. I suggest you try treating the symptoms first, by simply nibbling it, to see if it has any effect.

So What Do You Do?
If you get cramp at night, just keep a little pile of sea salt on your bedside table, and as soon as you start to feel the

cramp, put a little bit on your tongue and let it dissolve. Have as much sea salt as you like, and the feeling should disappear altogether.

If that works then try having a drink of sea salt before going to bed to see if you can sleep through the night with no symptoms. Once you've mastered that try increasing your daily amounts by adding it to food, or bathwater, so you don't need to have that drink last thing at night.

Of course, cramp doesn't only come at night, and for the times it could attack during the day, I suggest keeping a small amount with you. It's easy to do – simply keep some in a container in your handbag or in your car, and just nibble some whenever you feel like it, or when it's necessary, or, like John below, have it as a drink. Remember - once your mineral levels are back to normal any sign of cramp will indicate your mineral levels have dropped. This will probably be at times of stress in your life, and if that happens, you know what to do!

John, 77, says:
"I have suffered with cramp in the legs, body and arms for a long while. I have been on quinine tablets but unfortunately they do not seem to be able to do the job. I have been recommended to try salt, but not ordinary domestic salt: sea salt, with a little bit of water. And I have found that sipping it at night when I wake up with cramp, - because it wakes me up - clears it up very quickly. The only trouble is at the moment I am unable to find a little capsule to carry the salt around in!"

b) Headaches

An enormous number of people suffer from headaches, and one of the most common reasons we get them is a lack of minerals. Other common reasons include not drinking enough water, drinking too much alcohol, side effects of medication, eyesight problems, and stress. Other causes can be more serious, such as brain tumours. Some of us know what causes our headaches, and can relate them to lifestyle choices and triggers and know how best to avoid them. Other people need a trip to their doctor for a diagnosis. For many people, their particular problem is caused by a decrease in their mineral levels, often caused by stress, in one form or another. If you know that your headache is connected to your stress levels, or you are wondering if this might be the case, then adding some sea salt to your diet could make the world of difference.

How To Test it on Yourself

Next time you have a headache, as soon as you feel it coming on, put about an eighth of a teaspoon of sea salt into a mug and add some boiling water. Stir it, maybe adding cold water to taste, and then drink it. It's a bit like having a drink of yeast extract, or very weak chicken stock. It may taste uninteresting, or maybe slightly salty. If it tastes too salty to you, tip half of it down the sink, and add more hot water to make it weaker. You'll soon find the strength best suited to you. If you want more, or want to have a stronger mixture, then that's OK.

After about twenty minutes ask yourself if your headache is any different. If there is an improvement, then you know that a lack of sea salt and its minerals are connected to your headaches. Get used to altering the amounts of sea salt in the water to suit you. This could take a few weeks to really get to know, but as you get used to the drinks, you will soon be able to make yourself a drink that's just right.

If you find that after some testing, your headaches do not improve, then you know that your particular headache is not connected to your mineral levels. As we've discussed, lots of people have headaches, but many of them will have nothing to do with mineral levels.

If you find that minerals are connected to your headaches, I suggest introducing sea salt into your diet on a daily basis as that could greatly reduce the frequency and severity of headaches.

c) Hangovers

Hangovers are caused by drinking alcohol. The symptoms felt by someone the day after drinking can all be described as a hangover. Although these symptoms can include such things as feeling very tired, or grumpy, and being dehydrated, many people experience some type of headache. Medical advice would probably be to abstain from drinking alcohol in the first place, but for many of us having an alcoholic drink is part of our lives. One way of looking at it is that drinking any alcohol is stressful to the body, causing our mineral levels to deplete, and putting those minerals back should help you recover.

TOP TIP!

If you know you are going to be having a drink in the evening, then have a drink of the sea salt before you go out. Have another one before you go to bed, and another one next morning. You might be surprised at the results.

d) Migraines

Far more than just a headache, migraines can be so debilitating that sufferers may have to lie in darkened rooms for days at a time. Some people are so badly affected they will be unable to work or go to school. Others will have experienced a migraine on several occasions and have some idea what causes them. Some people will know that their migraines are connected to their stress levels, and if this is the case, then normalising mineral levels within the body may be of benefit. Common triggers for migraines are chocolate, cheese and red wine. However much you already know about your own migraines, I suggest you see if sea salt can help you.

For migraines we can take a two-pronged approach:

a) Taking the quick remedy, i.e. a sea salt drink as soon as you can feel the symptoms starting, and continue to take it, (i.e. have another drink,) if you feel it is helping. Don't worry too much if the drink tastes salty or strong.

b) You can take sea salt every day, and see if it lessens the frequency of attacks, by adding it to your food or putting it in your bath.

If you can establish a relationship between stress and your migraines, then sea salt may be of great benefit to you. If you have not established any reasons for your migraines, you could try the sea salt as described for stress-related migraines, and see if it helps. Remember, just because you haven't made a connection between stress and your migraine does not mean there is none. You may simply be unaware of the connection. It may be that there are so many factors involved with your particular migraines that working anything out is virtually impossible. If you record your migraines, start taking note of how much sea salt you are taking and see if there is any connection. If you see a health professional about your condition, discuss it with them as well, as two heads are much better than one!

Quick Fix: The Drink
1/8 teaspoon of sea salt in a mug of boiling water. Stir. Drink.

e) Nervousness and Panic Attacks

We can feel nervous for a wide variety of reasons, such as meeting new people, going to new places, or giving a speech. However, sometimes we feel nervous when there's nothing to feel nervous about. The first time this happens, it can feel quite weird, as your feelings don't really match up to what is happening at the time. For example, you may walk into a shop and feel a bit peculiar or uneasy, despite not having anything to feel uneasy about. You may be aware of your heart beating, or of your hands sweating. The feeling will pass and you will probably feel OK a bit later, and might not even comment on it. However if the same thing happens again a few days or weeks later, you will instantly be reminded that this has happened before, but once again you can't see any reason for feeling this way.

Some people will recognise that the above description is very similar to the first experiences of a panic attack. But for many, as there was nothing to actually panic about (by that I mean there was nothing scary and therefore no rational reason to panic), this occurrence can be very frightening. A similar type of situation is a hyperventilation attack. A hyperventilation attack is the same as a panic attack, but without any feelings of panic or worry. In both situations the body goes into 'fight or flight' – when it is preparing to react to danger, the heart and breathing rates increase, adrenaline is released, and because this puts stress on the body, minerals are lost. And as you are not about to start running or fighting, you can feel most peculiar. You may feel nervous, disorientated, shaky, or just plain weird!

Other people will describe their nervousness as a shaky feeling inside their body, as if all their organs have a slight tremor. Again, this is a worrying feeling. Often a trip to the GP or specialist will show that no physical problem exists.

Others feel as if they live on their nerves, or just feel very nervy, maybe always jumping a mile at a loud noise. They may notice that their friends often tell them to calm down, or tell them they seem very jumpy, or ask them what they are worried about. Often there is no answer to this as there really is nothing they're worried about – other than feeling nervous! Others feel the need to pace up and down the room. Just walking seems to calm them down and quell their physical symptoms.

All of the above examples are instances when our bodies lose essential minerals. In order to feel better we need to replace them.

So, whether you've got something to be nervous about or not, if you are definitely getting symptoms of nervousness, you may be able to remedy the whole situation by taking sea salt.

The instant remedy is to have a sea salt drink, or just nibble a bit of sea salt. However, I recommend increasing your daily sea salt levels to see if you can improve your nervousness in the long term.

Pamela, 50:
Despite having suffered ill health for over twenty years, one of Pamela's biggest problems is anxiety. Feelings of shakiness, nervousness and disorientation can sweep over her at a moment's notice, especially in shops, at events, and in restaurants. Her only way of coping with these in the past was to leave, go home and go to bed.

Pamela then started to use sea salt when she began to feel shaky or nervous. She found that by eating a small amount of sea salt (carried in a small, handy container in her handbag) she was able to carry on, and there was no need to go home.

She was generally unable to identify why she got the nervous symptoms, but soon started taking sea salt every day to keep her mineral levels up. Since taking sea salt daily, usually in food, she has had far fewer episodes of anxiety and has had to return home very rarely. Having a remedy that works has given her a lot more confidence and she now feels that she is able to tackle most things in life.

Quick Fix: The Drink
1/8 teaspoon of sea salt in a mug of boiling water. Stir. Drink.

f) Shaky Hands

When people notice their hands are shaking for no apparent reason, they can be worried that they have a serious condition, such as Parkinson's Disease. This can be very worrying, especially if a series of medical tests all turn out to be negative. As the person's hands continue to shake, for no clear reason, they can start to think there is something even worse wrong that the doctor hasn't yet realised, thus adding to their worry.

Does the Following Scenario Seem Familiar?

You feel as if you are shaking, so put your hand out in front of you so you can check to see if you are. Your hand may be shaking, perhaps so badly that holding a cup and saucer in one hand would be a bit dicey! Or maybe your hand isn't actually visibly shaking, but you can still feel the slight tremor within your own body.

The shaking may be caused by a lack of minerals or sea salt.

So What Do You Do?

Have one of the sea salt drinks or nibble some sea salt as soon as you become aware of the problem. Even if your hand isn't shaking, the fact that you are checking your hands is your own early warning system.

In my experience, the most effective remedy is having a drink of sea salt, which tends to relieve the symptoms in around 20 minutes.

Quick Fix: The Drink
1/8 teaspoon of sea salt in a mug of boiling water. Stir. Drink.

I recommend you increase your sea salt levels on a daily basis so that you don't get the shaky feelings in the first place. Once your levels are correct, you will probably only shake again when you are in a stressful situation. In which case, simply have some extra sea salt.

Mary, 76, says:
"I first noticed a slight shaking in my right hand when lifting a cup. Initially, I didn't think too much about it, but when it appeared to be happening a little more often than I liked, I decided to investigate what could be done. During a conversation with Sally, sea salt was mentioned as something which may be helpful. Upon doing a little research, I discovered that the minerals contained in sea salt may be of help, so I decided to explore the benefits of taking this.

After taking sea salt for a month, simply by adding it to food, there was a definite improvement and I have now been using sea salt for three months, during which time the improvement noticed previously has been maintained.

I shall most certainly continue to take sea salt on a regular basis and am most grateful to the author of this book for recommending it to me."

g) Anticipating a Big Day Ahead

When we have a big day in front of us, we can often feel nervous and anxious about it.

We could (amongst many other things) be:

in a competition
in the public eye
going to a wedding
going to a big party
going to a funeral
giving a speech
flying on a plane

Any one, or a combination of the above will mean that your body will be under higher levels of stress than normal.

You may start to feel anxious the day before the event and be slightly on edge. Or you could be feeling nervous. This can occur even if the event is an enjoyable one; something you've been looking forward to, such as a party. The golden rule is that if you are feeling slightly different, then your body may have already lost some minerals, and that mineral loss is what's contributing to your symptoms.

If you can relate to any of these things, I suggest taking some sea salt before you go, and carrying some with you, so you can add it to your food or drink later on.

You may find you feel OK for part of the day, but then find there's a dip and that you definitely feel worse. You may feel exhausted or emotional, or maybe you've simply got cold and wet. All of these will cause your body to lose essential minerals. If you have some sea salt with you, your remedy is at your fingertips.

h) Sleeplessness, Insomnia and Waking in the Night

Good sleep is when you fall asleep and wake up refreshed. There is nothing else involved. But for many of us, we fall asleep easily but find ourselves waking in the night, and then can't get back to sleep again. Others go to bed, but just can't fall asleep in the first place. For others still, their sleep is interrupted by the need to urinate.

Some people have a mixture of all these things, and all of them are classed as insomnia or sleeplessness. When we start to worry that we will not be able to get to sleep, or that we'll not get enough sleep, this adds to our daily stress levels.

A trip to the doctor describing our sleep problems can result in a battery of tests, and possible diagnosis that something is definitely wrong, such as sleep apnoea (see below). But for many people, there is no real solution, apart from sleeping pills or advice on diet before bedtime, such as reducing caffeine/alcohol levels etc.

All of these problems could be remedied simply by increasing our minerals, by taking sea salt. It's a much simpler solution than appointments with the doctor and tests.

One of the remedies for all these situations is to get your mineral levels back to normal by adding sea salt to your diet. In particular, have one of the drinks, as strong as you can take it, just before you go to bed. You may need to take sea salt every day to get your mineral levels back to normal before you see any difference in your sleep patterns. On the other hand, you may notice a difference on the first night.

i) Sleep Apnoea

There is also a condition called sleep apnoea, where the sufferer stops breathing whilst he/she is sleeping. He/she stops breathing, a small time elapses, then he/she takes a large breath, and continues breathing, all whilst still asleep. People with this condition are often tired throughout the day, and can fall asleep during daily activities. They often have a very poor quality of life. Some sufferers breathe in this way through the day as well.

One of the solutions for sleep apnoea is to wear a breathing mask at night. This is called a CPAP machine (standing for Continuous Positive Airways Pressure). Another solution is to restore normal breathing patterns 24 hours a day by learning the Buteyko Method. However, all people with this condition are under huge amounts of stress, as their fundamental breathing patterns are in need of constant checking. They will all benefit from normalising their mineral levels. This can be done by adding sea salt to their diets.

j) Frequent Urination

Some people find they need to urinate more often than they think is normal. Sometimes this affects them during the day, sometimes it only affects them at night, and for some, it seems to affect them at all times. There can be many reasons why someone needs to urinate more than normal. It could be due to illness, or because they're taking some kind of medication. However, most people have no idea that one of the symptoms of a diet too low in salt is the need to urinate frequently.

Some people think this problem is due to their age, (whatever age they are!), and that they will just have to get used to it, when in fact this simply isn't true, and can lead to people suffering with it unnecessarily.

People are often bothered by the fact they have to get up between one and six times a night, to visit the bathroom. This can really disrupt sleep patterns and affect someone's general overall health. Other people will find it embarrassing, when out with friends, that they have to visit the toilet more often than everyone else. In some cases, worrying about it can affect whether you want to go out with your friends in the first place.

If you come into any category above, and are bothered by the amount of times you need to urinate, then I suggest you try adding some sea salt to your diet. The first thing to do is keep a note of how often you need to urinate each day for a week. Also note if anything unusual or particularly stressful happened during that time. Examples of this would be doing more physical activity than normal, eating different foods from normal, having a big day out, sleeping badly one night, or being under any kind of stress.

Next, try adding sea salt to your food over the next week. You could also have one of the sea salt drinks just before you go to bed. Keep a record of the frequency of your urination and compare it to the first week's results. It may take time to work out how much sea salt you need to add to your diet, and, of course, you may need more when your body is under extra stress.

(If you are under your doctor's supervision for your urination, or any other medical complaint, then I recommend you discuss it all with your doctor and keep good notes, so he/she can assist you. This is especially important if you are on any medication of any description.)

k) Feeling 'Not Quite With It'

Do you ever feel not quite with it? There are many different names given to this odd feeling. I've heard people describe it as a dizzy feeling, of feeling peculiar, of feeling sideways, a swimmy head and a feeling of being unbalanced. You may feel a bit weird or odd. You may feel slightly disorientated or as if you may faint. These all have one thing in common: a normally healthy person suddenly feels as though they're not quite themselves. The strange thing is that it can happen at any time, and when not much is going on. So it seems very odd that you should feel so peculiar when there seems no reason.

There are many reasons why we can feel this way. We could be dehydrated, in need of food, or needing sleep. In the past you may have sat down and had a rest, or had something to eat or drink to help you recover. However, if your mineral levels have been low for some time, it could be due to them dropping even further. I suggest, as one of your solutions, that you try a sea salt drink and see if it restores you back to normal. You may find you feel better in as little as five or ten minutes. If the sea salt helps, then you know that weird feeling is connected to your mineral levels. I suggest, to stop this happening again, that you increase the amount of sea salt in your diet on a daily basis and see if that makes a difference over the long term.

Quick Fix: The Drink
   1/8 teaspoon of sea salt in a mug of boiling water. Stir. Drink.

l) Feeling World-weary

Sometimes we come home from work, or from visiting friends or family, or after a long day's shopping, feeling weary and needing a sit down and a rest. Many people will have a drink of water, a cup of tea or coffee, or a glass of wine. The caffeine, sugar, and alcohol in these drinks gives us a lift and, as we were possibly dehydrated, increase our fluid levels which may perk us up too.

An alternative to these drinks is a drink of sea salt. It will restore your fluid levels as well as topping up your mineral levels, which should make us more like ourselves.

Marion, 49:

Marion is a fit and active woman who works four days a week in a hospital. Having returned from a shopping trip with a friend, she felt weary and much older than her years. Her friend gave her a sea salt drink and Marion found that, within about 20 minutes, she felt hugely

better and ready for the rest of the day.
She now adds sea salt to all her meals,
and has the drinks when she is feeling
exhausted, or has returned from the gym.

Quick Fix: The Drink
**1/8 teaspoon of sea salt in a mug of
boiling water. Stir. Drink.**

m) Period Pain/PMT

Many women experience monthly changes to their bodies that can leave them feeling moody, exhausted, weary, craving unusual foods, and all manner of other symptoms. Thinking of the monthly cycle as a time of physical stress (where essential minerals are lost), it is easy to see why so many women have such problems. Adding sea salt to your diet can help by replacing those lost minerals. I also suggest increasing your sea salt intake when the symptoms start.

n) Teenage Girls

The teenage years are a very stressful time for girls, as they have to deal with the physical changes in their bodies as well as the emotional challenges of growing up. At times of such stress, getting adequate minerals into the diet is important, and this can easily be done with sea salt. If you have a teenage girl in your house and you are on the receiving end of mood swings due to hormones, see if she likes the sea salt drinks, and let her have unlimited access to sea salt.

o) The Menopause

Going through the menopause is a stressful time, both physically and mentally, in any woman's life for many reasons. Stress, as we've seen, can cause a drop in our bodies' mineral levels. Those minerals we lose need to be replaced.

It is interesting to look at the pills and potions marketed to women to help with the various 'female' problems. Many of the pills and potions you can buy to help you through the menopause contain minerals (for good reason!), but sea salt contains them too, and it's just as efficient a way of getting them into our bodies as well as being cheaper.

I suggest you try and get your mineral levels up to the correct levels throughout the month. You may find you need more minerals (in the form of sea salt) at certain times of the month. Excellent ways of increasing your mineral intake are bathing in some sea salt, having a drink of sea salt, or just adding it to your food.

p) Swollen Ankles

Cast your mind back to those old Victorian pictures of ladies bathing by the seaside. The ladies were usually fully clothed in frilly dresses, with frilly bloomers underneath. In most of the pictures, they were paddling with the sea up to their ankles. Why is this, you might wonder? For many, I'm sure it was because they liked a paddle. But maybe they knew something else: that paddling in salt water can help ease swollen ankles.

Swollen Ankles on Holiday

Many of us, especially women, suffer from swollen ankles when we go on holiday. While away, we might experience:

Hot temperatures, often completely different from home.
Inactivity, such as sitting on a coach, plane, or in a car for long periods.
Different hydration levels, as more water and fluid is needed in hotter climates.
Different foods, resulting in different mineral levels to normal.
Stress levels, good and bad, can be very different from home.

A good number of those suffering from swollen ankles complain that their symptoms are at their worst at the end of the day. The ankles can feel hot, puffy, and uncomfortable. One remedy is to paddle in sea water for about ten to twenty minutes. This may sound like an old wives' tale, but maybe those old wives knew a thing or two after all. The simple action of paddling in the sea can bring the ankles back to normal. This is most likely because the combination of activity, ie the walking, and absorbing minerals from the sea water through the skin, seems to remedy the situation.

If you are on holiday but not near the sea, or if you suffer from swollen ankles anyway, then soaking your feet and ankles in some water with sea salt in may just bring your ankles back to normal.

Swollen Ankles at Home

For those people who suffer from swollen ankles regularly at home, experimenting with soaking your feet in salty water is certainly worth a try. Whether you have swollen ankles periodically or daily, due to ill health, inactivity, or no known cause, you could create a beach in your home by trying the following:

Take a bucket or large bowl, or a foot spa, and half-fill it with warm water. Add some sea salt, and soak your feet and ankles for about 20 minutes.

Experiment with different water temperatures. The temperature isn't important – heat the water to a temperature you enjoy. Also experiment with different amounts of sea salt. Determine whether you need to immerse your ankles as well as your feet. You may find that this quite simple procedure is a solution to your problem. Although it can be quite messy, especially if you forget your towel, you may find it preferable to taking tablets and repeated visits to your doctor.

If you find the whole idea of soaking your feet in a bowl a bit of a chore, try adding the sea salt to your bath water and absorbing the minerals that way. All these methods will require experimentation, but there is no doubt that things can be absorbed through the skin.

Tuula and Judith:

Having spent at least four hours on a coach on holiday in Italy, Tuula and Judith had swollen ankles. They went for a paddle in the sea and within about 20 minutes their ankles had returned to normal.

q) Biting Fingernails

Many of us bite our fingernails, and if you are one who does you may wonder why you do it. This habit is often thought of as a symptom of nervousness, and often it is. However, there are many people who bite their fingernails who are not the nervous type at all and who, I imagine, would like to stop as it can be rather aggravating.

Another theory is that you have just got into a bad habit, and now can't stop, like chewing a pen whilst writing. And while this is often true, it does not account for why you started biting your nails in the first place.

If you look at your nails you will see they are very different from your skin. For a start they are much harder than your skin, even if they're flaky or weak. This is because the composition of the nail is very different to that of the skin.

The nail also has very little water content. In fact the nail is made up of different minerals. White spots on the nail, for example, can be an indication of too little calcium in the diet. (If you have ever had a full medical check-up by a doctor, he or she will have looked at your nails as part of his/her diagnosis.)

It is possible that you are biting your nails in order to obtain the required minerals for your body. There is an easy way to test if this is true in your case: add sea salt to your diet and see if the nail-biting stops.

r) Recovering from a Shock, an Asthma Attack, a Panic Attack, a Hyperventilation Attack, or any Fainting or Collapsing for an Unknown Reason

Have you ever had any type of collapse or attack? Did it take you some time to recover? Any of these episodes are a huge stress on the body and you may find sea salt an excellent remedy in the aftermath of such an incident.

i) Recovering From a Shock

Reacting to a shock is sadly a part of our lives, and the advice below is for everyday situations. It is not advice for the medical terminology of 'going into shock', so often seen on in medical dramas on the TV. Although many of the symptoms appear to be the same, they are two very different things.

Whenever we have a shock, whether it is physical (such as a car crash), or emotional (such as being told someone has died), our bodies can have a strong reaction by going into fight or flight immediately. You may feel the need to sit down, feel faint or lightheaded, or need a glass of water. Your face can go pale and you can feel very weak. Your hands may shake and you may find yourself becoming emotional, and fighting back tears. It can take ten or twenty minutes, or longer, to feel almost back to normal, and then even 24 hours to recover completely. None of this is pleasant, and you may feel a bit of a fool, especially if someone else has got involved, and is there to help you. They may be offering advice, such as suggesting a sugary cup of tea, or telling you to sit, or even lie, down.

I suggest you have one of the sea salt drinks as soon as possible, or have a hot bath with plenty of sea salt in it. Both of these methods will help your recovery.

ii) Asthma Attack

I have taught over 500 people with asthma to control their condition with the Buteyko Method, part of which includes having as much sea salt as is needed. An asthma attack consists of the constriction of the airways, making it difficult for air to be breathed in and out. Most people will carry a reliever such as Ventolin or Bricanyl with them at all times, and will take a puff when they feel their airways tightening. I always advise my clients that if they have any asthma episodes, whether or not they needed to take their reliever medication, a drink of sea salt would help settle them back down.

iii) Panic and Anxiety Attacks

Panic and anxiety attacks are very similar. Both occur when the body thinks it's in danger. Heart rate and breathing increase and adrenaline is pumped into the body to enable us to run away from the danger, or to fight it (this is often known as 'fight or flight'). And while it's an effective thing in nature, and would help us fend off an attacker or run from a charging bull, when it happens without there being any immediate threat, or as an overreaction to us worrying about something (flying, public speaking, travelling in a lift and driving on a motorway are four common examples), it can feel particularly scary and leave the sufferer feeling exceptionally drained afterwards, owing to the loss of minerals they've suffered.

A drink of sea salt should help you feel better. If you have many panic attacks, getting your mineral levels up to normal by adding sea salt to your diet should help. If you know you are likely to have a panic attack in the near future, for example, you are going in a lift today, then have extra sea salt before you go.

iv) Hyperventilation Attack (Read this section even if you think it can't possibly apply to you! You might be surprised.)

You may not have heard of a hyperventilation attack before. It is basically the same as a panic attack but without any feeling of panic or worry. For example, you may not worry about going up in a lift, or an aeroplane, but nevertheless, you feel ill. You may pass out, or feel as if you are going to die. You may have heard of the term 'panic attack' but because you don't panic, or are just not the panicky type, then you may never have read much about them.

You may have been diagnosed with 'hyperventilation attacks' but because you don't feel as if you are hyperventilating, or panting, then you may have dismissed the diagnosis. You may be aware, however, that you breathe through your mouth, or take an occasional large breath, cough a lot, feel as if you are not getting enough air, or that the air doesn't have enough oxygen in it. All of these can be considered chronic hyperventilation, (as opposed to acute hyperventilation) because you are breathing more than is required at any one time.

I suggest you try to get a better understanding of this condition. Try reading information about panic attacks, but just ignore the part about feeling and emotions. After all, who's got time to panic when you are sliding down the wall and passing out!

I suggest you have a drink of the sea salt to help settle you after any attack, and get your mineral levels back up to normal which should help you deal with them when they occur.

v) Fainting and collapsing

People tend to faint:

When it is too hot
When their blood pressure is too low
In hospitals
When they see blood
When they have a blood test
When they see needles
When they have had a shock
When they are starved of food
When dehydrated
When standing
After exercise
After feeling dizzy

Fainting is also known as blacking out, or passing out. Sometimes these episodes can be followed by seizures, also known as having a fit. While those who have suffered from frequent fainting will most likely have seen a doctor (and if you haven't, you should!), if you've only fainted a couple of times you've probably not. One reason for fainting is a lack of salt, which as you'll see, can be easily remedied. If you relate to any of this section, I suggest you discuss your salt intake with your doctor.

Although there is a lot of information about how to avoid high blood pressure, there is not much information in the media about low blood pressure. If your diet is too low in salt, the body compensates by reducing the amount of fluid. The consequence of this is that it is then harder to maintain blood pressure levels. This reduces blood flow to the brain and the central nervous system, which can cause fainting.

I suggest you add sea salt to your diet on a daily basis and see if it helps. If you

have a warning that you are about to
faint – for example, going slightly deaf,
having sweaty hands, feeling woozy,
feeling not quite all there – then try one
of the sea salt drinks as soon as possible,
or carry some sea salt in your handbag,
or in your car, and nibble some as soon
as possible.

Quick Fix: The Drink
1/8 teaspoon of sea salt in a mug of
boiling water. Stir. Drink.

s) Cravings Crisps, Nuts, and Other Salty or Spicy Foods

Some of us just love a packet of crisps, or tucking into a bag of nuts. Some people have a spicy meal once a week; perhaps eating out, or getting a takeaway. They see it as part of their makeup; part of their character, or as a treat they have earned after a hard week's work. In fact for some people, having a Chinese or Indian meal regularly is part of their social life.

Most of us would never connect the idea of our bodies requiring minerals with our desire for a spicy meal or a packet of crisps. In fact if you suggested to someone that their desire for a spicy meal was their body telling them they require more minerals and that they know that's where they can get them from, they would tell you that you are mad, and they just like crisps and nuts.

However, this 'desire' for salty or spicy foods is just the beginning of someone listening to their body, and carrying out its wishes. We may eat spicy foods, week in and week out, never being aware of what is happening.

Most salty snack food is made with processed salt, which does not have the mix of minerals our bodies require. The body is very clever, but when it needs salt or minerals it does not seem to be able to distinguish between processed salt and minerals/sea salt. Consequently it just craves something like crisps or nuts, especially as they are in a very handy pack at the supermarket, within easy reach and not hugely expensive, though recently some manufacturers are producing sea salt items such as crisps and even chocolate – so look out for those!

If the correct amount of sea salt is added to our daily diets it raises our mineral levels to their correct amounts, so we'll often find that we no longer think about crisps, nuts, or spicy meals. We will perhaps tend not to buy them at lunchtime, or no longer think about going out for a spicy meal, or once we are out for a meal, we may choose a different dish than before. It is as if, having got all the minerals required, our bodies are no longer steered towards the crisp aisle in the shop, or they no longer know beforehand what they want to eat before sitting down to a meal in a restaurant. We find that we just walk past the crisps and nuts, just like we often do past the washing powder, or newspapers.

Once you get used to having the correct levels of minerals in your body you will recognise the signs that you are deficient by your desire for salty foods, and when you're not, you won't be craving those fatty crisps, which is something your waistline will probably thank you for!

Asian foods tend to have a lot of different ingredients in them, many of them containing a large range of minerals, including foods which are not usually part of the western diet.

For example lemongrass contains calcium, copper, iron, manganese, magnesium, phosphorus, potassium, selenium, sodium and zinc. If you had previously been short of any of these minerals, a meal with lemongrass in it would satisfy your body's need for that mineral. There is nothing wrong with eating dishes with lemongrass in them, but once your mineral levels are back to normal, you may find you no longer want that particular dish.

Soy sauce, an important part of Chinese meals, is basically a salt sauce. You may be someone who claims not to eat salt at home, but love adding soy sauce to your Chinese meal. Again, this is just your body getting the minerals and salts from another place.

If you are home and are craving a salty snack, the easiest way to remedy the situation is to have either a sea salt drink, or just nibble a bit of sea salt.

Quick Fix: Nibble Some Salt

t) Stress, or Any Condition Made Worse by Stress

If you have been diagnosed with stress, or have any condition or symptom that is made worse by stress, whether listed in this book or not, then I suggest you add sea salt to your diet on a daily basis and see if you can improve your condition by adding minerals.

The following things are stressful to some. Some might surprise you!

computer screens
artificial lights
seeing family members
being in bright sunlight
when you get cold
getting wet
not having enough sleep
not taking in enough fluid
leaving too big a gap between meals
going to certain venues

having contact with certain animals
going in a lift

There are many different types of
stresses on the body. If you have
identified what makes your condition
worse, you may have started avoiding it.
For example, if you know going in a lift
makes you anxious and gives you shaky
hands, you may have started to avoid
lifts. This is fine for a while, but not
really a solution. One way to help
yourself is to add sea salt to your diet.
You may have some detective work to
do. You may find that just by adding sea
salt to your diet you are better able to
cope in stressful situations.

What To Do
If you know you're doing something
which will cause you stress in a few
hours' time, have some sea salt before
you go, either by adding it to your food
or by having one of the hot drinks. You

can also take some sea salt with you so you can top-up as required.

5
BUT WHAT IF I HAVE THESE SYMPTOMS AS WELL AS AN EXISTING HEALTH PROBLEM?

Many of us don't only suffer from some of the problems mentioned in the previous chapter, and it is likely that you may also suffer from a more long-term health problem as well.

You may have symptoms that are:

1 caused entirely by your long-term health problem and have nothing to do with minerals

2 caused entirely by a lack of minerals and have nothing to do with your long-term health problem

3 caused by your long-term health problem and made worse by a lack of minerals

In this next section we'll look at how adding unprocessed sea salt to your diet can help with longer-term and chronic complaints.

It may be that you have never analysed your symptoms to such a degree, and want to discover more. However, one thing's indisputable: the stress of a long-term health complaint will put additional stress on your body, which will deplete its mineral levels.

There are many people living with a long-term or chronic health problem, as well as other complaints, including:

Cancer
Brain tumour
Multiple Sclerosis
Mental health issues
Parkinson's Disease
Osteoporosis
Diabetes
M.E. /C.F.S.

Polymyalgia rheumatica
Heart problems
Liver or kidney problems
Breathing or lung problems
Stomach and bowel problems
Blood or circulatory problems
Living in constant pain
Joint problems
Skin conditions
Living with the result of injury or accident
Lupus

There are many more chronic problems, but as you can see, I have listed just a few.

All of these people are under huge amounts of stress, not only from the symptoms, but also from treatments, both of which may reduce the mineral levels in their bodies.

Consider the stress of the following:

Being unable to continue working or going to school

Being in constant pain

Being unable to walk unaided, maybe needing a stick or wheelchair

Being unable to continue with your hobby

Visiting doctors and specialists

Having numerous medical tests

Deciding whether to have an operation or not

Deciding which treatment to start

Having no choice as to your treatment or medication

Enduring long stays in hospital

Waiting for prognosis, or results of tests

Unable to go on holiday as waiting for results, or for treatments to start working

Cancelled appointments, tests needing to be done again, or your doctor not having the results yet

Knowing your health will not improve

Watching other people getting on with their lives

Enduring the side effects of medication

Starting yet another round of treatment; your life just going round and round with no end in sight

Each of the above puts additional stress on the body, either a physical, mental or emotional stress, and that is in addition to the physical stress and strain of the condition in the first place.

If you suffer from any of the above, adding sea salt to your diet could lessen some of your symptoms and make life a little bit easier. It will certainly help to replenish dwindling mineral levels, which will help you to feel healthier.

i) Already Taking Medication?

If you are taking any form of medication it is vital that you discuss your decision to take unprocessed sea salt with your doctor, specialist, or other healthcare professional. As there have been very few, if any, clinical trials into the taking of unprocessed sea salt, it is quite possible they will not have a standard answer for you. It is therefore a good idea to read all of this book and become knowledgeable about the whole concept of the benefits of taking sea salt.

When I used to teach people with asthma to change their breathing, I was often amazed at how little some people knew about the medication they were taking. For example, some were unaware that some of the asthma puffers contain steroids. Some were unaware their puffers contained adrenalin. Others were in a complete muddle about which medication did what. If you come into this category, even remotely, I suggest you get out all your medication and go through it all.

Check the following:

Its name
What complaint it is treating?
What is it meant to do?
Whether you are meant to take this medication on a regular basis, e.g. night and morning, or only take it when you have symptoms
Read the leaflet that comes with it
Ask yourself: do you take it as your doctor has prescribed, e.g. twice a day? Or do you take it in a haphazard manner?
Ask: are you presently increasing or decreasing the dosage? For what reason?
Are you doing this under medical guidance?

If you are vague about some of the above points, do not be surprised if your doctor is hesitant about you adding sea salt to your diet. On the other hand, your doctor might say it will not make any difference. However, if you are hoping to reduce some of your existing medication, solely because of the health benefits of sea salt, your life will be made a lot easier if your health professional knows what you are trying to achieve. Another point I would like to make is that if you have not been completely honest with your doctor about how much medication you have been taking (or lying about anything else for that matter!), now is the time to tell your doctor what you have been doing.

In my experience, people often didn't tell their doctor the exact levels of medication they were taking. They had either stopped taking it, never taken it in the first place, or taking a smaller amount than prescribed. For example, some people taking asthma medication were taking one puff of their inhaler night and morning, rather than the prescribed two. Or, they were taking far more over-the-counter medication than they were admitting to, for example, tablets for headaches. I think they were frightened that if they told their doctor what they had been doing, their doctor would refuse to help them in the future if they were ill. If this applies to you, go and see your doctor (perhaps taking someone with you for moral support), write down what you want to say, and as soon as you sit down in the chair in the consulting room, just start reading out loud from your script. Most doctors will just listen – after all, this is all new information to them – and the more information they have, the better they'll be able to help you. Once the record has been put straight, you can discuss the symptoms that are bothering you, and discuss the adding of sea salt to your diet. If your doctor seems a bit flummoxed, you can always say "so I thought I would add sea salt to my diet, and come back in seven to ten days to discuss how I'm getting on". You may need to explain the difference between sea salt and processed table salt, as defined in this book.

Some medications such as steroids (corticosteroids, not anabolic) may interfere with the mineral levels in the body. If you find you get more symptoms whilst on a certain medication, you may need to increase your sea salt intake whilst you are on the course of medication, then lower the sea salt levels once you have finished the medication.

ii) Blood Pressure Problems

For many of you, this will be the first page you turn to in this book. For some time now, we have been inundated with information about the relationship between salt and high blood pressure. The message has been that too much salt increases blood pressure to a point that is dangerous to our health. Whilst I do not disagree with the science behind this, it isn't the whole story. The majority of trials and studies on the subject, from which the information has been obtained, have been conducted using processed salt.

The fact is that a huge amount of the population are obsessed about their blood pressure and as a consequence have cut salt out of their diets, when in actual fact, it's only a small percentage of the people with blood pressure problems who need to be concerned at all.

At the National Heart, Lungs and Blood Institute Workshop on Sodium and Blood Pressure in January 1999 held in Maryland, USA, which examined evidence concerning the effects of sodium on blood pressure, it was stated that:

'Typically, studies to determine individual differences in blood pressure response to sodium intake have used a very low level of sodium chloride (10-20 meq/d) for several days followed by a very high sodium intake, provided either as a saline intravenous infusion or a high sodium chloride dietary intake over several days.'

As I am sure you can appreciate, there is a huge difference between a saline intravenous infusion, which is pure sodium chloride being administered by a drip into your arm at a certain rate, and taking sea salt, containing dozens of minerals, being eaten in various quantities, depending how much stress you have been under. (For more information go to www.nhibi.nih.gov/healthy/prof/heart/hbp/salt_sum.htm)

It is estimated that the majority of the general public are trying to cut salt out of their diet, whether they have been identified by their doctor as having high blood pressure or not. It is now common that if you offer someone any form of salt with their food, they decline, stating that they are watching their blood pressure. If you ask them whether they have high blood pressure, the answer is often 'no', but they are worried they might get high blood pressure in the future. The fact is that of all the people diagnosed with high blood pressure, only a small percentage actually have high blood pressure as a direct result of their salt intake. Other reasons for high blood pressure include being overweight, being on medication, or genetics.

Many people with blood pressure problems have a blood pressure meter and take readings on a daily basis. They may already be aware that such things as alcohol, certain types of food, or exercise, can affect their blood pressure. They may be on medication, and seeing their doctor on a regular basis. It is quite easy to alter one thing in your life, such as adding sea salt to your diet, and monitor how it affects your health. As sea salt is a great balancer of the body, some people may find that they are able to reduce the amount of medication they use, or come off it altogether.

I also recommend that those taking their blood pressure on a daily basis, at home with their own blood pressure meter, read the instructions as how to use the machine properly. A study in

Canada showed that most people did not use their meter correctly. For example, they did not sit for two minutes with their arm at heart level (i.e. resting on a table), and be silent for the duration. Most of the people in the study talked while they were sitting down, and were not silent at all! So read the instructions that come with the meter and make sure all your readings are accurate.

iii) Common Questions about Blood Pressure

Q. We are inundated with information about the connection between salt and raised blood pressure. What salt are they talking about?

A. Most clinical trials into the relationship between salt and blood pressure have been done using either table salt, which is highly processed, or a saline solution. Neither is a natural product and therefore is different from an unprocessed sea salt. I do not dispute any of the results of the clinical and medical trials; after all, they will have been carried out under very strict controls. However, they will also have been giving the same amounts of salt to each participant when, in my opinion, most people need different amounts of salt to each other, and they need different amounts each days. I'm not surprised there was a high level of abnormal activity in blood pressure readings when processed salt, which is an unnatural product, was given to a variety of participants. If you take the correct amount of sea salt for you each day, depending on what you are doing and how you are feeling that day, you tend to feel better rather than worse.

Q. I now take sea salt. Do I need to continue monitoring my blood pressure?

A. This is something you need to discuss with your doctor. I suspect he (or she) will monitor your blood pressure to the degree (s)he thinks necessary. Talk to them about it.

Q. My blood pressure is not the same every day. How will I know if taking sea salt has affected it?

A. Many things can affect your blood pressure, such as alcohol intake, exercise, being ill, eating different foods, taking some medications, even the amount of water you have consumed that day. Some people have abnormally high blood pressure readings in the doctor's surgery, but satisfactory readings when done at home. Some of these patients are given monitoring devices to wear for 24 hours to see what happens over a day, rather than just a few minutes. The human body has a variety of mechanisms to keep the body stable. It can alter its temperature, it can sweat, the hairs on the body can trap air for warmth, and the blood pressure can alter. These are all normal actions occurring in the body every day. So it is normal for blood pressure to alter throughout the day. Most people who take their own blood pressure with a monitor at home take it at the same time each day, to try to see if there has been any change. I suggest that if you have any of the symptoms in this book, check with your doctor first, then start adding a little sea salt to your diet to see if it can alleviate the symptoms, then return to your doctor, who can check your blood pressure again.

Q. I am fairly healthy, take regular exercise, eat a good diet, and am not overweight. My doctor takes my blood pressure once a year and says it is OK. I am worried that if I start taking sea salt my blood pressure will go up. After all, my doctor wouldn't keep taking my blood pressure if he wasn't worried about it, would he?

A. Your doctor is probably taking your blood pressure as part of an annual check-up rather than being concerned about it. If you are not sure, ask. If your doctor says your blood pressure is OK, then I see no reason not to believe him. I suggest you start adding sea salt to your diet to see if it alleviates your symptoms. If you are still worried, you could visit your doctor and have your blood pressure checked. If you're really unsure or are worried, simply ask your doctor why your blood pressure is being taken.

Q. I get terrible cramp in my legs after a long walk. I don't want to stop my walks as they are part of my social life, but the agony of the cramp is terrible. I am concerned about adding sea salt to my diet as I am worried it might raise my blood pressure and I might have to start taking medication.

A. A long walk, as opposed to short walks, can be a huge stress on the body, but I would describe it as good stress, especially if you take short walks on your own, at your own pace, and then do a long arduous walk; let's say once a month, with a walking group. On this occasion you will have to walk at someone else's pace, only stop for a rest when others do etc. There are lots of benefits of these long walks, especially for your social life, and the challenge of doing something a bit different. It is fine for you to add sea salt to your diet. Take a little extra before and after your long walk, and have one of the drinks before you go to bed after it. When you next see your doctor, tell them what you have been doing, he will probably check your blood pressure for you.

iv) Diabetes

If you have diabetes and one or more of the symptoms listed in this book, you may want to try adding sea salt to your diet to see if it improves your health. However, substantially changing any part of your life or diet may have an effect on your diabetes, so I suggest the following course of action.

First of all, you must have good control of your diabetes. By this I mean:

1 You must be monitoring your condition on a regular basis, usually daily, or as advised by your healthcare professional, and keeping good records.

2 The healthcare professional who monitors your condition must be satisfied with the way you take your medication, your record-keeping, and your response to problems, i.e. that you

make another appointment with him/her, and take his/her advice.

The above two conditions are important. If you are not sure if your health professional is satisfied with you, ask them!

So What Do You Do?

Start with the following:

1 Keep good records of your condition, writing down blood sugar readings, insulin taken, how you felt at the time and what symptoms you had, before introducing sea salt to your diet.

2 Visit your diabetes health professional and ask them if they are satisfied with your record-keeping, and ask them to help you over the next few weeks as you add sea salt to your diet to try to alleviate certain symptoms.

3 If your health professional agrees, add a small amount of sea salt to your food each day for a week. Do not have the drinks, or eat it on its own. Just divide your small amount into two or three very small amounts, and add it to your food, say for breakfast, lunch and evening meal. I do not like to prescribe an exact amount, because everyone is different, but keep it small as you can always increase it at a later date. Keep good records as before and return to your health professional.

Make sure that you have no added stress during the first week:

Don't add a different exercise routine into your week

Don't drink abnormal (for you) amounts of alcohol

Don't try this whilst on holiday

Don't start/ stop smoking

Don't start/ stop a diet

Don't start/stop a new job

or anything else that you think may alter your readings.

One of three things will happen

No Change
There is no change to the readings. From this you can deduce that a small amount of sea salt has had no detrimental effect on your condition. Note if any of your other symptoms (see section on symptoms) have improved. If you are enjoying positive benefits, you may want to try adding a little more sea salt to your diet, to try to alleviate some other symptoms. Simply increase the daily amount of sea salt, and repeat all the above again, returning to your health professional at the end of your second week.

An Improvement

The readings have improved, and/or you need less insulin. If this is the case, then you know that sea salt is a good thing for your condition. Continue to take the sea salt and discuss with your health professional what changes could be made to your medication levels in the future.

A Negative Effect

The readings have got worse, and/or you need more insulin. If this is the case, then you can deduce that sea salt is detrimental to your condition. Stop taking it straight away and in a few weeks' time consider trying again. Consider whether anything else during the week could have affected your condition.

v) Asthma and Other Breathing Problems

I have personally recommended over 500 people with asthma and other breathing problems such as emphysema, C.O.P.D. and panic attacks to add sea salt to their diets. These people came to me to learn the Buteyko Method, which I've mentioned in the introduction. Most understood that I was going to teach them to change their breathing, and most were surprised when I advised them to add sea salt to their diet. The Buteyko Method teaches people to do two things: to get their breathing back to normal by breathing approximately 5 litres of air per minute at rest; and to get their mineral levels back to normal by adding sea salt to their diets. There is not a set amount of sea salt to be taken each day. Each person discovers how much they require and alters the amount each day depending on need.

Virtually every single person I saw with breathing problems followed my advice, and saw an improvement in their health and wellbeing. I think there are two reasons for this: firstly, having any form of breathing problem, especially when you cannot catch your breath, is very stressful on the body, and secondly, many people with asthma are on some form of medication, which is itself stressful to the body as well.

Let us look at each of these in turn.

Stress number 1
Diagnosis

Being diagnosed with asthma, emphysema, or Chronic Obstructive Pulmonary Disease, is usually a lifetime diagnosis. To hear this can be emotionally stressful, whether you have a family history of similar conditions, and have seen what it does to your family members, or if it is a completely new and unknown condition in your family. And, as discussed before, the result of said stress is the reduction of the body's mineral levels.

Stress number 2
Learning about the condition
Learning about your diagnosis can be a steep learning curve. You may find information in books, leaflets, the internet, and anecdotal details from friends and family. Digesting the

information is an extra task you have to do, which is mentally stressful.

Stress number 3
Learning about the medication
Another steep learning curve is learning about your medication, finding out how it works, how it should be taken, and its side effects. Realising that you may be involved with this medication all your life can be emotionally stressful.

Stress number 4
Visits to the doctor, asthma nurse and/or specialists
For most people, visiting their own doctor may not be stressful, but once you start with visits to hospitals, asthma nurses, or specialists, the stress starts to add up. You may be required to breathe into apparatus, cough on demand, and all manner of things you are unfamiliar with. Walking down long corridors at

hospitals, finding parking places, travelling on unfamiliar public transport, and then being questioned on all manner of things, all add to the stress of these conditions.

Stress number 5
Living with the condition
Being unable to breathe is very frightening. It is also physically very stressful to the body, and will usually require some recovery time. People may find they feel shaky, or need to urinate soon afterwards. It can be enormously tiring to deal with it every day.

Stress number 6
Side effects from the medication
Common sense tells us that any medication will affect the body, and many will have side effects. Many people with breathing problems take steroid medication, either in inhalers (corticosteroids such as Pulmicort,

Becotide, or Flixotide), or in tablets (usually Prednisolone). Whether they are taking them every day, or after being prescribed for a few days, the side effects are numerous. The side effects of steroids include thinning of the skin, thinning of the blood, thinning of the bones, hastening the onset of cataracts, stunting growth in children, and localised problems in the throat area, such as thrush. Any of these side effects will be physically stressful to the body. (NB: Despite these side effects, DO NOT STOP TAKING YOUR MEDICATION WITHOUT DISCUSSING IT WITH YOUR DOCTOR.)

Stress number 7
Trying complimentary therapies/trying different diets
Some people will try a variety of complementary therapies to try and reduce the amount of medication they

need to take. Learning about each one, and deciding whether it works for you, is an added stress. Explaining this treatment to your doctor or asthma nurse is often stressful as their response cannot be guessed at, and the feeling of needing to keep your doctor or asthma nurse on your side often adds to people's stress levels.

Stress number 8
Realising that your life is changing
As time passes, and you continue to have problems, the realisation that your life will never be the same again can be emotionally stressful.

The above times of stress all add up, and for most people with asthma or other breathing problems, living under continual stress becomes a way of life, which means that their mineral levels are constantly being depleted.

It is no surprise that most people with breathing problems need a lot of sea salt. Even after a few days of taking sea salt, they often find that they have far fewer headaches, less cramp, sleep better, urinate less often, and are less nervous. Other minor symptoms seem to disappear as well.

So, as well as adding unprocessed sea salt to your diet, either by putting it on your food, taking it as a drink, nibbling on it or bathing in it, I also suggest looking into learning the Buteyko Method.

vi) Chronic Fatigue Syndrome, Myalgic Encephalomyelitis (M.E.)

The cause of M.E./C.F.S has not yet been found, and as such, we can only try to treat the symptoms, which are numerous, and commonly include fatigue, headaches, loss of short-term memory, and pain.

Let us look at the different stresses on a person with M.E.

Stress number 1
Feeling ill

For most people with M.E., they feel ill for quite a long time before they are diagnosed. They may have started with a virus which they haven't recovered from, or there may have been a slow onset of a variety of symptoms. This period is physically, mentally and emotionally stressful as most people do not know what is happening to them, and they are too ill and tired to do much about it.

Stress number 2
Finding a diagnosis
The process of being diagnosed with M.E. can be a long haul. Some doctors tell us that fatigue seen for less than six months is diagnosed as Post-viral Fatigue, which if it persists for longer than six months, it will be described as Chronic Fatigue or M.E. So by its very nature, diagnosis is not given for six months. During this time, people may have various blood tests to determine any other cause for the symptoms, which can be stressful, on top of enduring illness for such a long time.

Stress number 3
Diagnosis
It can be a huge relief to finally get a diagnosis. But discovering there is no

treatment, and not much prospect of getting better, is emotionally stressful.

Stress number 4
Work prospects
For those who've been forced to give up work, with no sight of a return, the stress increases. This may be coupled with a drop in income and encountering the benefit system. The financial implications start to hit home, and the life you had envisaged, with promotions, increased salary and daily interaction with work colleagues, seem a distant memory.

Stress number 5
Friends and family
People with M.E. are often amazed at the reaction of friends and family to their illness. It seems that because there is no plaster cast, medication, or treatments – nothing they can physically see and identify as an illness – some of their

friends and family think there is nothing wrong with them. Dealing with these reactions can be very distressing and adds to the stress of this condition.

Stress number 6
The length of the illness
Many people with M.E. are ill for years. I suffered from M.E. for over 20 years and experienced virtually everything in this section (although I would like to thank my family; they have been, and continue to be, very supportive). All the above stresses seem to happen again and again, so the stress levels continue to be persistently high.

Stress number 7
Trying different complimentary therapies
As there is no recognised treatment available for M.E., many people try different alternative and complimentary therapies. These can be helpful; many are not, and working out which help you and which don't can be stressful, and very expensive.

I have personally recommended to many people with M.E. that they add sea salt to their diet. Virtually every one of them has found it to be invaluable, and would not be without it. I also wonder if people with M.E. are unable to retain minerals in their bodies, as they seem to need such a lot of sea salt on a daily or regular basis. Conversely, it may be that M.E. causes such huge amount of stress on the body on a daily basis, that the need for minerals is on-going.

When Russell Stark (who was training me to become a Buteyko Practitioner) first recommended I added sea salt to my diet he suggested having as many as six mugs of the drink per day. Personally I find if I add enough to my food, I don't need to top-up with the drinks and I can tell when my levels are low as I crave salty food. So my advice would be for you to have as much sea salt as you feel you need.

I am going to take this opportunity to tell people with M.E./C.F.S. which therapy made me better. It is the Gupta Amygdala Retraining Programme: see http://www.guptaprogramme.com
If you have M.E. I recommend you take a look. It helped me to feel substantially better in about ten days, and I continue to use its techniques whenever I have any symptoms. I consider myself 90% cured. I still take sea salt everyday as well.

Anne, 61, says:

"Having had M.E. for very many years it is easy for me to do a 'before' and 'after' comparison in my health. Since regularly using sea salt I have noticed an immediate and significant improvement in my health. Also I often had bad headaches which have completely stopped now."

vii) Skin Conditions, including Eczema and Psoriasis

Eczema and psoriasis are skin conditions that affect both children and adults. The skin appears red and inflamed; it is itchy and uncomfortable. It can be flaky, and can look raw as well. The condition can be mild, often just affecting the hands. It can be moderate, affecting more of the body. Or it can be severe, affecting large parts of the body. While any of these conditions can be mildly annoying for some people, others may find the condition affects most of their lives. Treatments include creams that can be difficult to apply because they are thick and greasy, taking a course of drugs such as corticosteroids, and wearing certain clothes and bandages over the affected areas.

Some people have discovered that their condition is worse at certain times, for example in different climates, at different times of the year, when they eat certain foods, or when they are under stress. I suggest you read the chapter on the different types of stress as you may discover that your skin condition is more related to stress than you thought.

How Sea Salt Can Help

Having experience of dealing with numerous sufferers of eczema and psoriasis, I'd suggest either adding sea salt to your food, or putting some sea salt in a hot or warm bath and soaking for at least 20 minutes. I would try this every day for at least ten days to see if it improves your condition. In my experience, a lot of skin conditions tend to get worse for a few days before they get better, so don't panic if that happens.

Remember, for generations people with skin conditions have been soaking in various mineral-enriched waters around the world to try and improve their condition. At the Dead Sea for example, people coat themselves in the mud and wallow in the water for hours.

If you have ever noticed that your skin worsens when you are under stress, then all you may need is more sea salt in your diet, which can be taken orally, in a drink or with food.

You may be interested to know that during ten years of teaching the Buteyko Method, some of my clients had eczema or psoriasis. Most of them experienced a 'flaring up' of their condition in the first two to three days, then a huge improvement by the fifth day. I'd therefore suggest you learned the Buteyko Method and see if your condition can be improved by getting your breathing rate back to normal.

6
THE WORRIED WELL

Are the 'worried well' just lacking minerals? This modern-day label, depicting people who are worried about their health, but turn out to be healthy, is being applied to a growing number of people.

The scenario goes like this:

Following the latest advice on healthy living – such as eating five portions of fruit or vegetables a day, cutting out salt from their diets, getting lots of exercise, drinking less alcohol – an increasing number of people are finding they are not as healthy as they thought they would be. They have a succession of so-called minor complaints, such as cramp at night, shaky hands, and perhaps craving salty snacks. They don't believe their complaints are serious enough for them to arrange an appointment with a

GP, and often put them down to their age. They think it cannot be due to their lifestyle as they follow healthy living advice pretty closely.

So they believe that there must be something wrong with them. They consult their GP, eventually, who sends them for tests, only for everything to come back negative and they are proclaimed healthy. The trouble is, they are not actually that well. Maybe a few more symptoms have started, and the next trip to the GP starts everything off again.

Now look at it from the point of view of their mineral levels. Cutting out even processed salt will affect the body, and many vegetables grown today have very few minerals in them due the overuse of the soil, so even having their five a day isn't helping as much as they'd think. A chain reaction starts. A lack of minerals in the diet is a stress on the body. Symptoms start, such as cramp, or shaky hands, as I've mentioned before. As no more minerals are taken up by the body, the symptoms continue, and the situation gets worse. Medical tests (which can be stressful at the time) reveal nothing. This is stressful to hear, as the symptoms are still present on a daily basis. Believing they have some disease that the doctor has not yet found, or that medical science has still not discovered, is hugely stressful and compounds the problem.

You may not know if you have been labelled one of the 'worried well', but if some of the scenarios in this book are beginning to ring true, then you might have found your solution. Start by writing down all your symptoms, whether you have discussed them with your doctor or not. Include those things that are annoying and puzzling you. Add sea salt to your diet for one week and then return to your list and see if there's been any change.

7
CHILDREN

Children are under many different types of stress. They are physically growing, and they're constantly dealing with school and family, with timetables and clubs and practises, and with friends. Even playing is stressful, and that's before they've fallen over and grazed their knees!

You may regard it as part of growing up, but just as most parents try to help their children with stressful situations, one of the methods you can use is to make sure they have enough minerals in their food, by encouraging them to have sea salt when they are eating, whether at the table or in front of the TV, or with their homework. My advice would be to use sea salt when preparing and cooking their food, and if you have a particularly nervous child, you can always add sea salt to their bath water.

Children tend to take as much sea salt as they require. If their consumption of sea salt has increased you will know they are under some sort of extra stress.

When girls are teenagers there are many things they have to learn about, along with the other additional stresses – their changing bodies being the most obvious, but also having to learn to interact with a grown-up world. Teaching them about sea salt is important information for them as they learn about dealing with stress, and the benefits of minerals in their diet.

Anne, 61, says:

"My grandson Matthew, now aged seven, has, from being a toddler, asked for sea salt, which he loves to eat on its own. I let him have it because I realise

that his body must be craving minerals
and I know how pure sea salt is."

8
HOW TO TAKE SEA SALT

As you'll see from this chapter, adding sea salt to your diet is very easy. What you'll need to remember is that the amount of sea salt you'll need will differ from person to person, so what I suggest you do is:

1 Make a list of your symptoms (even if they're not mentioned in this book). Record how often they occur and how severe they are when they do. Do this for a week before you begin taking sea salt.

2 Add sea salt to your diet in one of the ways I suggest in this section and, still keeping your symptom diary, record the frequency and severity of your symptoms again.

For most complaints, I'd suggest beginning with the sea salt drink or adding sea salt to your food. If your symptoms improve slightly, then try increasing the amount of sea salt to see if you can alleviate the symptoms altogether.

As I explained earlier, the amount of salt you'll need will depend on you as an individual. One of the great things with sea salt is that you will be able to tell, without any expensive consultation, exactly how much you need. It will also differ on different days, depending what you are doing during the day, and how much stress you are under.

After a few weeks you will be able to recognise which of your symptoms are connected with your mineral levels, and which have no correlation at all. As a general rule, any symptoms or conditions made worse by stress should improve after adding sea salt to your diet.

i) Cooking With Sea Salt

Most people will remember seeing mothers and grandmothers, or fathers or cooks, adding salt to most dishes they made, adding it as they cooked and tasting as they went. And they did this for a reason: adding salt to food brings out the flavours. But salt's not just a great ingredient because it makes things taste better, or because it prolongs its shelf life – if it's unprocessed sea salt it's a way of getting essential minerals into your body as well.

If you would like to try adding sea salt to your food, one of the easiest ways of doing so is to go back to the old fashioned way of cooking with salt. Keep a pot of sea salt by the cooker and add it to all savoury dishes. Most people start off adding just a little, afraid that the dish will taste too salty, but in my experience, this very rarely happens. As time goes on, you will get used to how much sea salt you need to add. One thing that is almost bound to happen is that your food will taste even better as salt is known to bring out the flavour of the food.

Easy ways of adding more salt to your food

1 If making spaghetti Bolognese, add a little sea salt to the water that the spaghetti is cooking in, and add a little to the Bolognese sauce as it cooks.

2 Add a little to the water when boiling vegetables such as potatoes, carrots, cabbage, broccoli etc.

3 Add a little to homemade sauces and soups.

4 Sprinkle it over roast meats in the oven.

5 Sprinkle it over roast potatoes in the oven.

ii) Sprinkling It On Your Food

You may think it strange that there is a section in this book about such a simple action as sprinkling salt onto your food. It is necessary because many of us nowadays don't sit at a table to eat, so we don't have easy access to salt once we are eating, and even if we do sit at a table, there may not be salt within reach.

Sprinkling sea salt onto your food is one of the easiest ways of adding minerals to your diet. All you need to do is sprinkle a bit onto your food, to taste. You can always add a bit more later, if you need to. The alternative is to put a little pile of it on the side of your plate, and dip your food into it as you go along. Some people wonder if they can have too much sea salt with this method, and the answer is no, as your taste buds will indicate whether you have added too much.

Some suggestions

1 Just sprinkle a little sea salt on such items as tomatoes, cheese, or eggs on toast – it tastes great!

2 Sea salt tends to fall off chips so why not just dip the chips in some salt on your plate?

3 You can sprinkle sea salt into any dish you stir – soup, stew, bolognese; even salad. You might be surprised how much better it tastes, AND it'll be doing you good!

You may also find that adding sea salt to your food will mean that you don't need to add quite so much of those sauces and condiments – soy, ketchup, etc. all contain salt (just have a look at their labels). By adding the pure product, i.e. unrefined sea salt, you may find your desire to add other sauces diminishes. This is your body requiring less processed salt as it's now getting the real thing.

The same applies to yeast spreads, such as Marmite, Vegemite, and Bovril as well. After using unrefined sea salt, the need or desire for these products may wane.

You may like to keep a record of what your body is craving, needing or just desiring and see how it alters. You may be surprised!

Even though you may have already added salt to your food while cooking, you may be surprised at yourself for wanting to add it to your food after it's been served. Do not be too alarmed at this. Listen to your body, and if you would like more, than have a bit more. Often you will have sea salt left on your plate at the end of a meal. The fact that there is some left over indicates that you stopped adding to your food as you were eating your meal. It is a good sign; a sign that you are tuning into your own body's need for minerals.

iii) The Sea Salt Drink

"The Quick Remedy"

When anyone suggests drinking sea salt, most of us will have memories of gulping large mouthfuls of sea water by mistake whilst on holiday, or being forced to drink salty water in order to make them sick. Neither makes you think that a drink of water with sea salt in it will be a pleasurable experience – but you might be surprised! Taking some sea salt in a hot drink is one of the quickest ways of getting minerals back into your body, and more and more people are trying it and finding that, actually, it's quite all right.

Here's what you do:

Put about an eighth to a quarter of a teaspoon of sea salt into a mug, and add boiling water. Stir it. (If you don't like to take your drinks piping hot then feel free to add a drop or two of cold water.) Have a little taste. If it tastes too strong, or too salty, just tip half of the mixture out of the mug, add more water, and try again. When you're happy with the taste just drink it as you would a mug of tea or coffee.

It should taste unremarkable, or even bland. You may find this puzzling, as you will be aware that you have just put sea salt in your drink and expect it to taste disgusting, or like sea water. I used to tell my clients that if they can't taste it, their bodies must really need it. If it becomes unpalatable part-way through, just stop: it's your body telling you that you've had enough.

Experiment with different strengths until you arrive at one that you like, and can easily drink. Sometimes you may want a stronger mixture, sometimes a weaker one. It can take a couple of weeks to really tune in to what your body requires.

One way of looking at it is to recognise that if your body is quite happy to drink sea salt dissolved in water, then it must really need it! You will notice, on some occasions, that it tastes really salty. This is your body telling you that it doesn't need any more minerals at that time, so there is no need to drink the rest of it. In fact, your body will not want to drink it.

Children under 12 hardly ever like the drinks, and often seem to make a big fuss if you try to get them to drink it, so for them I'd suggest using other methods, such as adding sea salt to their food or letting them nibble it. However for teenagers, especially girls, having a drink of sea salt whenever they want can be very useful as their bodies change.

Having a drink of sea salt is often the fastest way to alleviate headaches, hangovers, cramp, shaky hands, nervousness, and after a shock. After just 20 minutes you may feel hugely better.

Some people have between one and six drinks a day, substituting it for tea or coffee, and keeping their mineral levels topped up. You can also add sea salt to a variety of drinks, such as fruit juice, fruit cordials, tea or coffee.

Some people worry that they will have too much sea salt – after all, we are bombarded with information telling us that salt's bad for us. You just need to remember that the salt you are taking contains all the correct minerals, and your own body will be able to work out how much salt you need, so don't panic, just try and tune in to how much your body wants at any particular time. You may find you always want a drink of sea salt first thing in the morning, or you want different strengths of the drink at different times of the day. You may require different amounts on different days, depending on your circumstances and what stress you may have been under. You can't have too much sea salt as your body will tell you to stop by making it taste too strong. But remember, tuning in to your body can take a few weeks.

Once you have gained confidence with the drinks, and realise they help with a particular problem, you may decide to have a strong-tasting drink, just to get the minerals into your body as fast as possible. As long as it solves the problem, this approach is fine.

Quick Fix: The Drink
1/8 teaspoon of sea salt in a mug of boiling water. Stir. Drink.

TOP TIP: HAVE YOUR FIRST SIP STANDING BY THE SINK. IF IT'S TOO SALTY IT'S OK TO SPIT IT OUT.

iv) Nibbling It

Some people just like to eat sea salt neat. They can tell when they want some, and just nibbling a bit makes their symptoms go away in double-quick time. I've noticed that children especially seem to like this method, and will ask for sea salt, the same way they will ask for a glass of water. Don't let this alarm you, just think that if your child asks for sea salt, and then eats it neat, he/she must simply require more minerals. I suggest adding more sea salt to their food, and you should notice they will ask for it less often as their mineral levels get back to normal.

Some people, if they are in a situation where they know they need some minerals – for example when their hands are shaking – will just nibble a bit of sea salt, and put up with the strength of it, rather than take time to boil a kettle and make the drink. It seems that, when sea salt is absorbed through the mouth, it works very quickly. The sea salt drinks can take up to about 20 minutes before a difference can be seen in symptoms, but nibbling it can take substantially less time. Once you have established that your symptoms can be reduced by having some sea salt, you may be less fussy about how you take it.

v) Bathing In It

For hundreds of years people have travelled to places such as Harrogate, Bath and Buxton to 'take the waters'. These spa towns, having mineral springs close by, marketed themselves as places to go to rejuvenate one's health. This was no fad, nor just a fashionable place to be seen. It wasn't something that was all over within a year, or even a generation. This business was so successful that these towns became important places and even cities. For these towns to have prospered for so long, their customers must have returned on many occasions, and recommended them to their friends and families. For that to occur, they must have felt that their health had improved whilst they were there.

In 1760, Doctor Richard Russell recommended the use of sea water for enlarged lymphatic glands. He wrote 'A Dissertation on the use of sea water in the Diseases of the glands. Particularly the Scurvy, Jaundice, King's-Evil, Leprosy and Glandular Consumption.' He preferred sea water to inland mineral waters. He moved to Brighton, and started a successful medical practice based on sea water being good for you.

So there is a correlation between bathing in waters containing minerals and feeling an improvement in health.

There are many reasons why we like bathing in the sea, such as freedom of movement and fun. But added to this is a feeling of wellbeing, which could be due to the minerals in the sea being absorbed through the skin. There is the added bonus of breathing in air that is high in minerals, and this may be why so many people go for a walk along the promenade, apart from watching the world go by and being seen in the latest fashion! The high levels of minerals in the air and sea persuades people, especially the elderly and retired, to move to the seaside. This exodus to the seaside has been a regular occurrence for generations (in fact it all started with Dr Russell), and today some seaside towns have an older than average population.

Daily sea bathing is not feasible for most people in the UK, so bathing in water which has minerals in it is the next best thing. The minerals can be absorbed by the skin quite easily, especially if the water is warm or hot. A few years ago it was thought that nothing could be absorbed through the skin, but now even drugs are administered by absorption through the skin in the form of patches.

Epsom salts have been used for decades. They consist of magnesium, sulphur and oxygen, a blend which is known as magnesium sulphate. Over the years, claims have been made that bathing in Epsom salts can aid all sorts of ailments such as asthma, preterm labour, cerebral palsy, boils, carbuncles, abscesses, acne, genital herpes and shingles. Once again, a mixture of minerals are linked to good health.

In addition, for those people who hate the taste of salt and cannot even tolerate a pinch of sea salt in their food, then bathing in it is an easy way to absorb minerals. Bathing in a sea salt bath is also highly recommended to women shortly after childbirth. After all, people have been adding bath salts, bubble bath, bath oils etc. to their baths for years.

If a full bath is not an option, just try soaking the feet in a bowl of warm/hot water with sea salt in it. Again, this is something that people have done over the years, and can be pleasurable.

Debbie, 41, says:

"On my midwife's advice, after each of my three children were born, I took a daily bath in sea salt to help my body recover after having had numerous stitches."

What To Do

Just add half a handful of sea salt and stay in the bath for about ten to twenty minutes. You may get the urge to urinate during that time. This could be a sign that you have absorbed enough minerals.

For those looking after an elderly relative, and who supervise their bath time, just throwing in half a handful of sea salt is an easy way to ensure they are getting some minerals each day/week.

If you have a skin condition and normally shy away from adding anything to your bath water, just try a small amount for a few weeks, and see if it makes a difference. You may find your skin condition flares up at first, but then settles down, and is better overall. Generally, bathing in sea salt is an easy way of ensuring you get some minerals on a regular basis.

TOP TIP: THROW A HANDFUL OF SEA SALT INTO A WARM BATH. STAY IN IT FOR 20 MINUTES

9
TYPES OF STRESS

Stress comes in many forms, and while some of them might surprise you (you might not even realise you had them!), they all have a significant effect on our bodies. We often hear of people being 'stressed' or 'stressed out', and we often associate stress with people working for long hours in offices, or with working mothers, coming home to care for their children after a hard day's work or other high-pressure situations. Often we see these people as fitting a huge amount of activity into their day. But the reasons for stress are many and varied and go far beyond this. To understand the relationship between stress and salt, we need to understand the exact nature of stress on the body.

There are lots of different types of stress, and they all have the same effect on the human body.

They can be separated into the following categories:

Physical Stress

Walking up a steep hill is physically stressful. It feels harder than walking on the flat. It can make us quite breathless, and we may need to stop for a rest. It can increase our heart rate and we can be aware of our heartbeat; something we rarely notice normally. Even something as simple as walking while carrying heavy shopping is a physical stress on the body, as it is a lot harder than simply walking.

A gym session will be stressful. Activities such as running on a treadmill, or using the equipment, are all a stress on the body.

Having a medical procedure such as an operation, or someone taking a blood sample, is also physically stressful. The skin being punctured, or cut open, will have an effect on our breathing and heart rate.

While none of these things are bad for us, and some have their benefits, each one involves the body being under physical stress.

Mental Stress

Mental stress can come in many forms. It involves using your brain as opposed to your body, to do something you find difficult. Having to sort out your VAT return, or fill in a form from the Inland Revenue or the Health Department, are examples of things that are mentally taxing or stressful. For some people, anything that involves numbers will be taxing; for others, anything that involves writing pages of information will be stressful. Mental stress can be as simple as trying to remember something.

All these things, and hundreds more, are mentally taxing and stressful to the human body. Often they are things that have to be done on a daily or weekly basis, and depending on your strengths and weaknesses, some will be more stressful than others. They may also be easy to do in the morning, let's say, when you are fully awake and ready for the day, rather than trying to do them in the evening, when you are feeling tired and in need of a rest. You may remember thinking, 'Yes I should fill out that form, but I'm too tired to do it now, as I might get it wrong.' So you wait until you are more able, say, next morning. This shows that even quite easy jobs can be mentally stressful.

Emotional Stress

Emotional or psychological stress can be short- or long-term. For example, splitting up with your partner, or nursing a sick pet, would be short-term emotional stresses. Caring for people with mental health problems, such as your ageing parent, who requires your attention on every single thing in their life, is an example of long-term emotional stress. Having to deal with unpleasant people at work, or unwanted attention from your employer, are other examples of emotional stress. Often, this kind of stress will be due to a series of small, irritating things which, individually, are easy to dismiss. Or you may feel other people would not be as irritated as you are, and that maybe you're overreacting and should be better able to cope. You may feel you have difficulty coping with whatever is going on around you. All these things are emotionally stressful and take their toll on the body.

Environmental Stress

The two most common environmental stresses are pollution and the weather.

Pollution

Pollution causes big problems for the human body; so much so, that there are Acts of Parliament such as the Clean Air Acts to ensure that the whole population is breathing unpolluted air. Another Act, The Health and Safety at Work etc. Act (1974) ensures the environment in which we work is clean and safe. Similar legislation has dealt with drinking water and other potential problems such as the dismantling of factories, food safety, car exhaust fumes etc. Should anyone be subjected to pollution, the reaction on the body can be immediate, for example, accidentally inhaling car fumes causes you to react by coughing and spluttering. Some reactions can take years, such as with the inhalation of asbestos fibres. Both of these are stresses on the body, with visible results.

The Weather

The weather, if it is very hot or very cold, is also a huge stress on the body. Also a change in the weather, which is very common in the UK, is stressful. Our climate can be described as having all four seasons in one day. This means that your body's temperature control mechanism has to work harder to keep your core temperature equal throughout the day. This mechanism also has to work hard if you go from a cold environment, such as being outside, into a much warmer environment, such as a centrally heated house, or department store. Often this is remarked on: we'll say things like, 'Isn't it hot in here?' Some people with long-term health conditions, such as arthritis, experience a worsening of their condition when the weather changes.

People don't often consider that their body is under stress in such circumstances, but it is.

Family Stress

Just being part of a family, whether you live with them or not, can be stressful. It can be different for each family member. A father who watches his sons play football every weekend may be under very little stress, but a working mother who might have to make sure all the football kit is clean and ready, week in and week out, might have a different tale to tell!

And, of course that extra stress isn't only down to children. Partners and financial worries play their part too. And with many of us living longer that we used to, many people find themselves being a part of the sandwich generation, with elderly parents to care for as well as young children. We can feel as if we are being stretched in two directions as we make decisions and care for three generations. Another example are working mothers, who, working during the day and caring for children the rest of the time, never have a moment they can call their own, and often spend their time just trying to catch up with all the jobs that need to be done. They often feel guilty as they feel that what they accomplish isn't ever good enough, either at work or as a parent.

Christmas brings about an annual stressful time, as family members who maybe don't see each other for most of the year all converge in one house to have a 'perfect' time. The film industry has made many films about such a time, most showing bizarre behaviour by normally quite reasonable people. The films show whole families under stress for a short period, but for some people, they are under continual stress throughout the year.

Financial Stress

Being unable to afford all you would like or need can be described as financial stress. Being under threat of redundancy, or on a short-term contract at work, can add to financial worries.

This may mean you are unable to risk changing jobs and have to stay where you are. Often financial concerns tend to affect whole families as long-term plans such as holidays, new cars, moving house, or house renovation fall by the wayside as money is needed for essentials.

School Stress

Many school children feel stress as they start a new term, have a new teacher, are sitting exams, being bullied, or can't keep up with the pace of the lessons. They may find it all too easy, be bored, and looking for something else to do. With younger children, stress may manifest itself as complaining of a tummy ache, or headache when it is time to go to school. Some children miss lunch, and find it hard to concentrate during the afternoon. Some get lost in larger school sites and wonder if they will ever find their way to their next lesson. Although all these things can be seen as a normal part of growing up, they are all examples of a child being under stress.

Work Stress

Stress at work is not always a bad thing. Some of us like working to deadlines, and some even thrive on it. Others like to work in the public eye, where their every move is scrutinised. But for many people, working is just a way of earning money, where it can become stressful when we are asked to complete too much work, or complete it too quickly, or take on someone else's job as well as our own. We may be aware that we may lose our job, or only be on a short-term contract and need to start job-hunting again soon. For some, the actual job may be OK, but the other people in the office/factory may make things unpleasant. A long or tiresome journey to work, such as overcrowded trains or difficulties in parking the car, can all be regarded as work stress. For many of us this is constantly with us and part of our lives.

Good Stress

Stress is not always bad for you. Think of someone running fast on a treadmill at the gym. While they will be doing this to improve their health and fitness levels, their body is definitely under stress. Consider someone anticipating a party: they may be looking forward to it, but even the good stress may have increased their heart rate.

For many people with health conditions that are made worse by stress, they may find they experience just as many symptoms anticipating a party as they do going outside on a cold winter's day.

Smoking, Alcohol, and Illegal Drugs

While some of us might not be able to fathom why people would inflict these things on themselves, many do, and in so doing, put additional stress on their bodies. Smoking, for example, is so harmful to health that there are government health warnings on packets of cigarettes. But thousands of people still smoke, and the stress on the body of pollutants and tar etc. result in such conditions as emphysema, heart disease, and cancer. People who smoke are physically under stress every day as they have to deal with cravings and side effects, as well as other people's disapproval.

Alcohol can be a conundrum. Where a small amount can help people feel relaxed and cheerful, too much alcohol can result in liver problems, alcoholism and in some severe cases death.

Illegal drugs create stress on the human body. Some will have various short-term 'good' effects similar to alcohol (otherwise there would be no reason to take them in the first place!), but in the long term, virtually all the stresses are detrimental to the body. People often are undernourished, and lead a life addicted to a substance that has no benefits to their body. They are under large amounts of physical stress as well as the mental and emotional stress of being dependent.

Medication (Prescription Drugs)

People who take medication daily are under stress every time they take it. This is not to say it is a bad thing to take it; rather that, in addition to the illness requiring the medication in the first place (which is a stress in itself), adding a substance to the body will cause a reaction.

Being Overweight or Underweight

Being overweight presents many health problems. Imagine someone struggling to walk up a hill because of the extra weight they are carrying. They may be huffing and puffing and red in the face. They are putting their bodies under stress as they walk up the hill. However, being underweight also presents problems. This may be due to an unsatisfactory diet, or just the fact that when they are ill, and lose weight through, say, a week of eating practically nothing, it can take a long time for the weight to restore back to normal.

Are You Under Stress?

Sometimes it is easier to recognise stress in other people than to observe it in yourself. So take a little time now to consider the following:

What short-term stress you have been under recently?

What symptoms did you display?

Did you do anything to recover, such as sit and have a rest, have a drink, have an alcoholic drink, have a cigarette, visit the toilet, or collapse in a heap?

What long-term stress have you been under in the last six months?

With a bit of hindsight, what symptoms have you been displaying?

Are you still displaying these symptoms?

How have you been dealing with this stress?

Look ahead to next week – what stressful situations will you have to deal with?

Are you already displaying symptoms such as worry, dread or irritation?

It is easy to dismiss stress as just part of our lives. Indeed, for many of us it is part of our life, and we just get on with things and ignore it as best we can. We tend not to think we are ill, but think we just have to put up with symptoms such as headaches, cramp, urination in the night, or poor sleep patterns. Often some of us assume it is just our age, and part of growing older. Many of these symptoms have become so common that if you tell someone else about your symptom, they tell you they have it as well, only much worse!

This can make us feel that we won't bother the doctor with such a trifling problem, as his surgery must be full of people with much more severe problems than ours. However, your own problem has not been solved and now that you have discounted seeing your doctor, you may have no other recourse than to put up with it for the rest of your life.

Luckily, one of the easiest solutions to your predicament is within reach. Just by adding sea salt to your food, bath water etc. you can eliminate your annoying symptoms for good.

10
ABOUT SEA SALT

i) What's In Sea Salt?

As I've said, may times, in this book, unprocessed sea salt contains many minerals. But which minerals are in it? As I've already said, that can depend on where the salt has been harvested from. But for those of you like me, who'd like to see actual data, here's a list of exactly what was present in sea salt harvested from Anglesey in 2009:

Hydrogen
Chloride
Sodium
Magnesium
Calcium
Potassium
Bromine
Carbon

Nitrogen
Strontium
Boron
Oxygen
Silicon
Fluorine
Argon
Nitrate
Lithium
Rubidenum
Phosphate
Iodine
Barium
Molybdenum
Uranium
Vanadium
Arsenic
Nickel
Zinc
Krypton
Cesium
Chromium
Antimony
Neon

Selenium
Copper
Cadmium
Xenon
Aluminium
Iron
Manganese
Yttrium
Zircon
Thallium
Tungsten
Rhenium
Helium
Titanium
Lanthanum
Germanium
Nobelium
Hafnium
Neodymium
Lead
Tantalum
Silver
Cobalt
Gallium

Erbium
Ytterbium
Dysprosium
Gadolinium
Scandium
Cesium
Promethium
Samarium
Tin
Holmium
Lutetium
Beryllium
Thulium
Europium
Terbium
Mercury
Rhodium
Tellurium
Palladium
Platinum
Bismuth
Thorium
Indium
Gold

Ruthium
Osmium
Iridium
Radium
Radon
Francium
Actinium
Protactinium
Niobium
Praseodymium
Ruthenium
Tellurium
Helium
Sulphur

Quite a list, I'm sure you'll agree!

ii) Where Does Sea Salt Come From?

To understand sea salt we need to know where it comes from in the first place. You may remember this from geography lessons at school, with diagrams of rain, earth and sea illustrating rainfall and evaporation. But if you're anything like a lot of the people I've taught over the past few years, you could probably use a reminder. So, let me remind you. . .

When it rains, the water seeps into the ground and then runs into streams, which run into rivers, which end up in the sea. The earth is made up of a huge variety of different soil types: different clays, rocks with different mineral content, peat bogs etc.

The composition of the world's surface is so complex, some people spend all their lives studying it. Put simply: the water, running over and through the various surfaces on the earth's crust, picks up different minerals from different areas as it flows. This water runs into streams and rivers, and ends up flowing into the sea. Once there, tides and currents mix it together, and other matter – fish, crustaceans, plankton, sea flora and seaweed – are added to the mix as well. So we can think of the sea as a huge mixture of minerals and water.

This mineral mix can be extracted from the sea in a variety of ways, and once the water has been removed, the remaining solid matter is called 'salt'. When you look at salt in this way, you can see that sea salt is, in fact, a mixture of minerals.

The content of the mixture will vary depending on its location. The sea salt from the salt pans of Lanzarote, for example, has a slight pinkish colour due to the high incidence of shellfish in its waters, whereas salt extracted from Wales is much whiter. There are also seasonal variations, as sea creatures die and produce different levels of calcium as their shells break down and disintegrate at a certain time of the year.

The sea contains a huge variety of minerals – about 84 different ones – and it is thought that the mineral mix within the sea is virtually the same as the mineral mix within the human body. Evolution states that humans came from the sea, and it is therefore not surprising that our mineral makeup is so similar.

If you have ever swum in the sea you will know that once back on dry land, if you don't rinse the sea water off, your skin can feel itchy and even look a bit scaly. This is because some of the salt from the sea has stayed on your skin, and the water has evaporated. If you flake off a bit of the scaly stuff and taste it, it will taste of the sea, and taste salty. What is on your skin is unprocessed sea salt.

Unprocessed sea salt contains a mixture of minerals, and as we know, the human body requires a mix of minerals, often in very small quantities, to keep it functioning as it should and to keep us feeling healthy. It makes sense to add unprocessed sea salt to our diets.

iii) How Do We Get Salt Out of the Sea?

For years, many coastal areas of the UK extracted salt from the sea. This can clearly be seen by the number of place names with the word 'salt' in them, such as Saltcoats in Ayrshire, Saltfleet and Saltfleetby in Lincolnshire, and Salthouse in Norfolk. In some of these places, the old salt workings can still be seen.

In hot climates, sea water is fed into lagoons and left for days in the sun for the water to evaporate. At a certain stage, when it becomes more of a 'mush', it is drained, with gravity's help, into smaller lagoons. It continues to be dried by the sun, and eventually the salt crystals separate out. The salt 'mush' can be lifted out of the lagoon with a spade, left to dry some more, then put into bags to be sold.

If you have travelled to other countries, you may have seen the 'salt pans'. In Lanzarote, for example, part of the tourist trail includes looking over the huge salt pans from a viewing point above the bay. Tourists look down over a patchwork of rectangular salt pans, each one silvery-pink in tone; each different to the next, and each changing its colour as the sun moves across the sky. As the sun reflects off the different salt concentrations in the various pans, it is a spectacular sight.

Although the evaporation method was used in the UK, the average daily temperatures are too low for this to be done commercially. Therefore other methods are generally used. Boiling sea salt under pressure and then letting the water cool allows the salt flakes to be separated, and lifting the visible flakes

from the cooling water is quite easy.
Once again the salt is dried, this time in
ovens, and the salt can then be packaged
for storage, or used straight away.
Although this method is not such a feast
for the eyes as the salt pans of
Lanzarote, some sea salt producers are
open to the public, and make an
interesting visit.

iv) The Difference Between Sea Salt and Rock Salt

About 250 million years ago, Britain
was close to the equator and covered by
a shallow, inland sea. It was surrounded
by desert. As the land drifted northwards
(we call this continental drift), some of
the salt beds were left exposed and
disappeared. Others, though, were buried
– and that's what we call rock salt,
which is in fact sea salt which has lain
buried for many, many years.

In the UK, and in Cheshire especially, the salt is mined underground, mainly for gritting the roads. The reason you are not advised to eat this type of rock salt is that different companies add de-icing agents to make it more effective at dissolving snow and ice. It also has to be able to flow properly out of the gritters. It is this type of rock salt that is found in roadside grit bins, and is not for human consumption.

Like sea salt, rock salts from different parts of the world will contain different minerals, or different concentrations of minerals. One brand of Himalayan rock salt is described as pink; the pinkish colour coming from the specific mixture of minerals.

Any rock salt marketed for human consumption will contain minerals in the same sort of quantities as sea salt, and can be used in the same way as sea salt. If you use a particular rock salt, but you still have some of the symptoms listed in this book, it may be worth trying a different rock salt or try a sea salt and see if you can eliminate your symptoms that way.

v) Is the Sea Salt I've got at Home The Right Stuff?
(The difference between unprocessed sea salt, processed sea salt, and processed salt)

You may be surprised to know that the salt you buy to put on your food may be totally unprocessed and natural, or it can be highly processed and, consequently, two very different products. Even products that are described as 'sea salt' and found in the salt aisles at supermarkets may have been processed and are not acceptable from the point of view of this book, as they don't contain the minerals we need.

All sea salt essentially comes from the sea, but what happens to it next is the determining factor. Once harvested, it can either be sold for human consumption immediately, or it can be processed.

Unprocessed Sea Salt

This is the category of sea salt that I recommend, because this salt contains numerous minerals which are beneficial to us. The companies that sell this type of sea salt are very proud that their products are unprocessed. A quick glance at the packaging will contain the following type of information, so you can clearly see what it is. Look for the following phrases:

Coarse sea salt (The word 'coarse' means it has not been crushed.)

Small pieces of shell, stones and pits may be found in the product (Do not be put off by this!)

Grey moist sea salt (If it is grey it can't have been washed!)

Hand harvested (i.e. not by machines.)

French salt marshes (The French area of Guerandais produces a grey sea salt that can be bought on the roadside in France, in large bags.)

Harvested using old methods of draining and withering (The fact that old methods are being used means it has not been mechanised. Withering means drying under the sun.)

Certified to be without chemicals

Certified to be without anti-coagulation treatments

Unbleached (Although some unprocessed sea salts are white, many are grey.)

Natural

Ancient and clean

Natural minerals and trace elements

Whole, not refined

Free running without chemicals (Obviously no anti-caking agents used here.)

Left to naturally crystallise

Scooped off by hand

Fruit of the ocean, the sun and the wind

Hand harvested

Traditional methods

Guaranteed not to be washed or refined

Free from additives

Naturally rich in magnesium

Source of calcium and iron

Over sixty naturally-occurring trace elements

Often this type of sea salt may not be in the salt aisles at the supermarket. You may have to go further afield.

Other places to look are:

On the internet (search for any of the words above)
Local health food shops
Farmers' markets
Local fish shops
Wholefood aisles in supermarkets
Home baking or home cooking aisles of supermarkets
'Products from around the world' sections
Luxury food sections
'Exotic' food sections
Gourmet food sections
Food fairs
County shows

Don't be put off if it looks a bit dirty, or says it's for baking, or for fine dining. Just read the packaging. Also have a look at the grains. You should be able to see that they all look different, somewhat flaky, as if they have come straight from the sea. How well do you think these flakes would pass through machinery? Your answer should be that they would block it.

There may be a difference in price between the different sea salts, but they are not necessarily more expensive than table salt.

Salt from the Dead Sea is often marketed solely for use in the bath or foot spa. It may not be labelled suitable for human consumption. This may be because the mineral mix is not quite correct for us humans, but it may just be that it can't be certified as clean! If that is the case, do not eat it! Some Dead Sea products are labelled as having been 'tested, approved and licensed by the Israeli Ministry of Health', but only for bathing in, not consuming.

Processed Sea Salt

There are many products that are described as 'sea salt' but have been processed in some way. They may have been processed to make them run freely in a salt cellar, or bleached to make them white. The amount of residual minerals will differ with each product. These products are a sort of halfway house. Unless you research them you won't know what's in them. You may also find that if you try to use this sea salt to help alleviate your symptoms, it won't work because the mineral that you particularly need has been removed. The individual pieces of salt often look very similar to each other, or can look shiny, as if they have been polished.

Many people assume they have the correct salt at home, when in fact what they have is processed sea salt. When teaching, I often suggested my clients show me. When we tipped a small pile onto the table we could see that all the grains were identical. They were all very shiny and they looked polished. When compared to an unprocessed, natural sea salt, it was easy to tell the unprocessed one as the grains were uneven looking, flaky, and some pieces were a lot bigger than others.

Processed Salt That is Not Described as 'Sea Salt'

This is the salt found in most people's homes. It is white, free-flowing, and all the grains look identical to each other. If you pour some into a little pile, you can easily imagine it flowing through machinery in a factory. If you look at the packaging it will probably just list sodium and chloride as its ingredients. The packaging may also say that it includes an anti-caking agent. If you taste it, you may notice it tastes unpleasant, and may make you wince – you can understand people not liking the taste of salt if that is their only experience of it. This salt is used in most packaged, pre-prepared, or fast food that comes from factories. This is the salt I want you to avoid.

vi) Dehydration Salts

Dehydration salts are a mixture of salts, sugar and water. They are used for children and adults with diarrhoea and are a commonplace remedy in the western world. They are also used in the developing world, especially at times of famine and disease, such as cholera. Packaged in sachets, they can be easily administered by people with very little training. They have saved lives all over the world.

When someone has diarrhoea, they lose fluids and minerals. Undigested food rushes through the body so fast that minerals cannot be absorbed by the intestines. The remedy is to take a mixture of salts and sugars. The dehydration salts contain sodium, chloride, glucose, potassium and citrate in a formula recommended by health organisations across the world.

If you have had an upset stomach and would like a quick remedy, a sea salt drink might well do the trick. It may just replace some lost minerals and help you feel a bit better. A sea salt drink can also be used after exercise. Try different concentrations of the drink to find out which you prefer.

vii) A Little Information on Mineral Supplements

We know that minerals are essential for our health and for our bodies to function as they should, and we also know that unprocessed sea salt is an inexpensive and efficient way of obtaining them. But sea salt isn't the only way – many people vouch for taking mineral supplements.

You may have some mineral supplements in a drawer in the kitchen or medical cabinet in the bathroom. Now is the time to get them out and look at them.

First things first, check all the date stamps and remember to throw out any that are past their use-by date. You may wonder how a mineral supplement could be past its sell-by date; after all, it has probably been in the ground for decades, if not centuries. The answer lies with the company that makes them. They will have processed the original mineral in some way, and if they say don't eat it, then I recommend you don't!

The packaging on mineral supplements tells us that the minerals are needed for 'bone health', 'body functions', 'blood formation', and 'enzymatic reactions'. If we did not know this, we would not buy them, and the companies that make them would go out of business.

Minerals either come from the land or the sea. They may have been mined out of the earth, or extracted from the sea. Either way, they are a natural product. However, most mineral supplements will have been processed in some way. They may have binding agents to hold the tablets together, and/or glazing agents to make them shiny and easy to swallow.

There are two types:
1 A single mineral, such as iron, calcium, or zinc
2 A multi-mineral (which may also contain vitamins)

Single Minerals

Some people will take a single mineral supplement because they have had a consultation with a doctor and have been recommended to take a supplement for a certain condition. If this applies to you, then continue taking it. If you suffer from any of the symptoms in this book, then talk to your doctor about taking sea salt, and whether you can reduce your intake of the single mineral supplement.

Other people have ended up with a hotchpotch of single mineral supplements that they once thought would be good for them, but have forgotten to take. If you haven't noticed much difference, I suggest they are not particularly useful for you.

Multi-minerals

The packaging on multi mineral supplements sometimes suggests that they are for people with an insufficient dietary intake. However many people take them everyday, even though their diet is fine.

If you look at the list of minerals on the packaging, you will notice a long list of minerals and details of how often to take them. Notice it will be 'daily', or 'three times a day', which is the same number of times most people eat a day. It would be just as easy to add sea salt to your food three times a day.

The minerals are present in tiny amounts, sometimes referred to as 'trace' minerals. This is similar to the amounts found in sea salt.

One problem of taking a daily mineral supplement is that you consume exactly the same amount of each mineral each day. This would be fine if you did exactly the same activities each day, ate exactly the same foods, drank exactly the same fluids, and were under the same amount of stress. People today don't tend to live like that. They tend to be under different stresses each day, and consequently their bodies will require different amounts of minerals. If you change to sea salt, you will start to self-regulate how much you need each day. With a mineral supplement, if could be difficult to know if you are taking too much, and you may have ended up over-prescribing.

If you are already taking a multi-mineral, and have none of the symptoms in this book, I suggest you try sea salt as it will be cheaper to buy.

If you are taking a multi-mineral, but still have any of the symptoms in this book, I suggest you change to sea salt and see if it gets rid of your symptoms.

Once you start taking sea salt, you probably won't need to spend money on mineral supplements at all.

11
HOW SALT IS SEEN TODAY

Over the last few decades there has been a huge shift in food production in this country. In the 1960s and 70s, most food was bought from a local butcher and greengrocer on the high street, housewives fed their families with a variety of dishes, and food fashions often only stretched to such things as a roast on Sundays, fish on Fridays, and cold meat in lunchtime sandwiches. Such things as fat content, vitamin levels, food miles, and locally sourced food were not even an issue, and rarely discussed.

In more recent times, more food is produced in factories and transported across the country. Whereas people used to work in factories producing steel, car components or cotton cloth, people are now working in factories producing butter, lasagne, or pizza. People buy much of their food in supermarkets, where 'choice', it seems, has become the most important consideration.

With this increase in mass-produced food has come an interest in safety of the food, with all factories having some sort of quality control, both on the ingredients as well as the finished product. Added to this is the labelling of food, with all the ingredients listed, and as time goes on, more and more aspects of food production are being discussed, such as the original source of the ingredients.

The media has become involved in all aspects of food – it's all over the television, radio, newspapers, and the internet. Whole programmes are dedicated to food, not just explaining how to cook something, but aspects of animal husbandry, documentaries on school dinners, and horror stories of cruelty to battery chickens.

And while we're talking about food, I think it's important to mention the horror stories we've all seen about many foods containing too much salt. Salt is added to food for a variety of reasons, including to increase shelf life and taste. With regard to taste, 20 years ago salt and pepper were always provided on the table, either at home or in a café or restaurant, and you were able to add them both to your food as you ate. It was sometimes seen as an insult to the chef if you added salt to your food before tasting it, but once tasted, no one had a problem with anyone adding salt or pepper to a dish they had prepared. If you consider a typical family sitting down to a meal in the 1960s, it is likely that they added different amounts of salt to their food. Someone working on the land all day (and therefore under a lot of physical stress) may want more salt than someone who had been sitting in an office all day.

Compare that with meals today. So-called convenience foods are designed to be heated up and eaten. There is no real preparation, so no one to complain if you add some salt! Food is often eaten at a work desk, while walking along the street, or while we sit and watch the TV. Often there is no salt (nor pepper) within reach. Many people have lost the skill of adding salt to their food.

We are also being told to reduce the salt in our diets. I find this quite bizarre, as everyone is different, and different people need different levels of salt in their diet. It is very rare to see anyone in the mass media telling us to increase our salt levels, or to even just keep them the same.

So I think it's worth remembering why salt should, in many instances, be added to food and that actually, it's done with good, sensible reason.

The biggest problem is that most people don't realise the huge variety of mineral mix in the different types of salt, from just two minerals (sodium and chloride) in refined, processed table salt, to up to 84 minerals in an unprocessed salt. I have often heard it said that 'salt is salt', and that there's no difference between salts, but I hope you can see the difference and start adding unprocessed sea salt to your diet today!

12
FREQUENTLY ASKED QUESTIONS

For all questions about sea salt and blood pressure go to Chapter 5, part iii).

I thought I shouldn't have too much salt. Isn't increasing the amount I have bad for me?

We all need salts and minerals. We need different amounts depending on what activities we have been carrying out. For example, someone who's been active all day will need more replacement salts than someone who's been watching them. There is a difference between fully mineralised sea salt and table salt. Table salt only contains two minerals, sodium and chloride. Sea salt contains up to 84 minerals, and that's what we should be having. Our bodies will tell us when we've had enough as the salt will simply taste too salty.

Where should we get the salt from?

Sea salt can be purchased in health food shops, farmers' markets, specialist food centres, and online. Some sea salts have been processed and probably do not contain the full range of minerals. A good way to tell the difference is to put some on the palm of your hand and look at the grains. If they look all the same or polished in some way, then they have probably been processed. If the grains all look different, and look as if they have come straight from the sea, then they are probably OK. Most grey sea salts have not been processed and are OK, even though they might look a little unappetising.

How much salt can I have?

You will probably need different amounts on different days, depending what you have been doing. Start with a small amount and see if you can get rid of your symptoms with just a little sea salt.

What shall I tell my doctor?

That you are adding unprocessed sea salt to your diet/bath to increase your mineral levels and to alleviate your particular symptoms.

I don't like the taste of salt. How can I take it?

Many people don't like the taste of processed salt. It can make you wince! However, unprocessed sea salt tends to taste different. Try a few different sea salts and see if you can find one that suits you. If you can't tolerate any in your food, just use it in the bath.

Do you recommend one type of salt as opposed to any other?

As long as it is an unprocessed fully mineralised sea salt, it should be fine.

What is the difference between rock salt and sea salt?

Rock salt is salts and minerals that have been trapped in the ground. It is usually mined out of the ground. Sea salt is the salts and minerals found in sea water. It has to be extracted from the sea and dried out.

My dad is elderly. Is he too old to have salt?

No. Anyone can add sea salt to their diets.

Can you give it to children?

Yes! Children often like the taste, and they need minerals for growth.

What are salt tablets that soldiers eat in the desert?

They are mineral supplements to make up for the lost minerals and salts due to excessive sweating due to the heat.

How can I tell if the salt is for human consumption?

It will say so on the packaging.

13
CASE STUDIES

Case study 1
Steve, 50, The Chimney Sweep

Having been a chimney sweep for over 20 years, Steve found that although he loved his job, his body was beginning to object. In particular he found that he got a lot of aches and pains, and felt stiff in the morning, which he put down to the abnormal positions he had to get into when cleaning awkward chimneys. He did a little exercise, had a fairly healthy diet, and didn't smoke.

After hearing about sea salt, he started to add a handful to his bath every day. Rather unusually, Steve has two baths a day to get rid of all the soot and grime.

Within a few weeks he noticed that he wasn't so stiff in the mornings and his body didn't ache. He decided to do some exercise and started running. At first he couldn't run very far, but a year on, he runs five and a half miles regularly. He is delighted with his progress and continues to add sea salt to his bath.

Case Study 2
Joe, 49, The Archer

Joe, 49, works as a stonemason, designing and building fireplaces to order. Over six foot tall and strong, he enjoys archery at weekends. With his height, strength and a calm manner, he did well at his hobby and before long started entering competitions, eventually becoming so proficient that he now represents his county.

Joe found that if the weather was warm all day, with no rain, he was likely to be placed near the top of the rankings. However, if it rained and he got wet and cold, his scores went down and his shooting deteriorated, resulting in a lower rank. He also knows that his body is under stress every time he competes – he is under mental pressure to do well, as well as the physical stress of the actual shooting. On cold, wet days, he found that he was tired and that his concentration levels were poor, and his hands were shaky.

As well as making sure he keeps dry and warm, Joe now adds sea salt to his food on the day of a competition, and has sea salt drinks as often as he needs them. He now no longer suffers from the tiredness, loss of concentration, and shaky hands and his scores on cold, wet days are now the same the ones he achieves on warm and dry ones.

Case Study 3
Mary, 72, The Ballroom Dancer

Mary, 72, has always been fit and active, and now in her seventies, attends two ballroom dancing classes a week. She and her husband have trained hard, and over the years gained a variety of medals and awards. Most people meeting her would think there was nothing wrong with her health, and consider her fortunate to be so active at her age. But Mary noticed a problem with her hands. She noticed they were shaking. At first it was just a little tremor, but sometimes her hands were so shaky she had difficulty carrying a cup of tea without spilling the contents into the saucer.

Mary visited her doctor, fearful of hearing the words 'Parkinson's Disease', but thankfully the doctor reassured her that that was not what she was suffering from. He conducted a few tests, but nothing showed up positive. With nothing more to be done she was resigned to having to put up with it for the rest of her life.

When Sally saw her hands shaking, she recommended Mary started taking sea salt, either in food or as a drink. Within a few days Mary's hands were back to normal, with no shaking visible. This continued for some months and Mary was able to hand out cups of tea to whoever wanted one. One day, Sally noticed that Mary's hands were shaking again. She asked Mary why this was. Mary said she had been away for three weeks visiting her daughter, and had simply forgotten the sea salt. She started having sea salt again that day and all the shakiness went away, just as it had before.

14
A FEW FINAL WORDS

I hope you've found this book useful and that unprocessed sea salt becomes both a daily addition to your diet and a useful remedy to have at your fingertips. If you are adding sea salt to someone else's diet (or bath) on a regular basis, please tell them, so they can account for any changes in their condition.

I wish you good health. Remember to take your sea salt with you when you go away!

If you have enjoyed this book then you might also like my other book, How To Breathe: The Symptoms if You Get it Wrong, and How to Fix It.

THE END

ACKNOWLEDGMENTS

The author would like to thank:

Russell Stark for training me to be a Buteyko Practitioner, for all his help and expertise, and for giving me a drink of sea salt when I was ill.

Jennifer Stark, for advancing my training as a Buteyko Practitioner, for trusting me with her students and trainees, and answering all my questions so completely.

All my family and friends who stuck by me and encouraged me to keep going with the book.

The Bollington Writers' group, who listened week in and week out to page after page about sea salt, for their helpful advice and encouragement.

All my Buteyko Clients who asked me to write a book in the first place.

Moolesto Perdomo Medina, for permitting access to the salt pans in Lanzarote.

Dr Konstantin Pavlovich Buteyko, who shared his knowledge of normalised breathing patterns with the rest of the world.

Alexander Stalmatski who brought the Buteyko Method to Australia and the UK.

David Lea-Wilson and his staff from Anglesey Sea Salt Company, who have answered my questions and allowed me to use their data.

Nik Perring, my editor, who helped me at every opportunity, and brought this book to fruition.

All the people who gave permission for their stories to be told in this book.

26102539R00130

Printed in Great Britain
by Amazon